Chest Wall Tumors
A Comprehensive Review Book

Foreword
SHAILENDRA KUMAR

SHUBHAJEET ROY
MEHUL SAXENA
ANURAG RAI

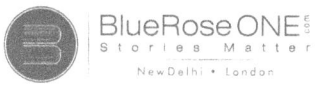

BLUEROSE PUBLISHERS
India | U.K.

Copyright © Shubhajeet Roy, Anurag Rai, Mehul Saxena 2024

All rights reserved by author. No part of this publication may be reproduced, stored in a retrieval system or transmitted in any form or by any means, electronic, mechanical, photocopying, recording or otherwise, without the prior permission of the author. Although every precaution has been taken to verify the accuracy of the information contained herein, the publisher assumes no responsibility for any errors or omissions. No liability is assumed for damages that may result from the use of information contained within.

BlueRose Publishers takes no responsibility for any damages, losses, or liabilities that may arise from the use or misuse of the information, products, or services provided in this publication.

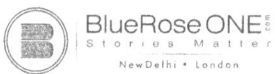

For permissions requests or inquiries regarding this publication,
please contact:

BLUEROSE PUBLISHERS
www.BlueRoseONE.com
info@bluerosepublishers.com
+91 8882 898 898
+4407342408967

ISBN: 978-93-5989-777-6

Cover Design: Sadhna Kumari
Typesetting: Pooja Sharma

First Edition: February 2024

Dedicated to:

To all our families, teachers, students, and most importantly the patients from whom we learn a lot.

Authors

1. **Shubhajeet Roy**

   MBBS Final Year Student,

   Faculty of Medical Sciences,

   King George's Medical University, Lucknow

2. **Dr Anurag Rai,** *MBBS MS MCh (CTVS)*

   Associate Professor, Department of Thoracic Surgery,

   King George's Medical University, Lucknow

3. **Mehul Saxena**

   MBBS Second Year Student,

   Faculty of Medical Sciences,

   King George's Medical University, Lucknow

Foreword

It is with great pleasure and admiration that I pen the foreword for this distinguished compilation on chest wall tumors. As a seasoned practitioner in the field, I have witnessed the evolution of thoracic oncology, and this book stands as a testament to the ongoing commitment of the authors to unravel its complexities.

The pages that follow reflect not only a deep understanding of the subject matter but also a keen awareness of the dynamic nature of chest wall tumor management. The authors, under the guidance of their mentors, have meticulously woven together the threads of clinical experience, research findings, and the nuances of patient care.

In navigating this resource, readers will embark on a journey that transcends the traditional boundaries of medical literature. The interdisciplinary approach and holistic perspectives presented within these chapters exemplify the collaborative spirit required to advance our understanding of chest wall tumors.

As a senior colleague, I commend the authors for their dedication and commendable efforts in producing a work that will undoubtedly serve as a cornerstone for those navigating the complexities of thoracic oncology. May this book inspire a new generation of clinicians and researchers to further enrich our understanding of chest wall tumors and, most importantly, enhance the care provided to those affected.

Prof Shailendra Kumar, *MBBS MS MCh (CTVS)*

Professor and Head, Department of Thoracic Surgery,

King George's Medical University, Lucknow

Preface

In this comprehensive review book on chest wall tumors, we embark on a journey through the intricate landscape of thoracic oncology. As we navigate the pages ahead, we delve into the nuances of diagnosis, treatment modalities, and the evolving understanding of these complex lesions. This compilation serves as a valuable resource, bridging the gap between medical literature and practical insights, offering clinicians, researchers, and students a curated exploration of the challenges and advancements in managing chest wall tumors.

Within these chapters, expert contributors unravel the clinical intricacies surrounding various chest wall tumors, shedding light on the diverse histopathological entities and their implications for patient care. The synthesis of current research findings and clinical experiences provides readers with a nuanced understanding of the diagnostic dilemmas and therapeutic considerations in this specialized field.

The preface is a gateway to an illuminating voyage, where the convergence of medical expertise converges with the relentless pursuit of knowledge. As we embark on this intellectual expedition, may the pages ahead inspire curiosity, foster collaboration, and ultimately contribute to the collective wisdom that propels the field of chest wall tumor management forward.

We extend heartfelt gratitude to the contributors of this book, whose dedication and tireless efforts have sculpted this invaluable resource. Behind every insightful contribution lies the unwavering support of families, whose patience and encouragement enable the pursuit of academic excellence.

To the esteemed teachers and mentors, your guidance has been the compass navigating the authors' intellectual journey, shaping their understanding and fostering a commitment to advancing medical knowledge. The debt of gratitude extends to the students who have played a vital role in the authors' growth, challenging ideas, and propelling the discourse forward.

Last but not least, our deepest appreciation goes to the patients—the true catalysts for medical exploration. Their resilience, trust, and shared experiences form the bedrock upon which this body of work stands. It is with profound thanks that we acknowledge the symbiotic relationship between medical practitioners and those whose lives they touch.

Date: *26th December, 2023*

Place: *King George's Medical University,*

Shah Mina Road, Chowk,

Lucknow-226003, Uttar Pradesh, India

Acknowledgment

We acknowledge the efforts of all the contributors of our book: Prof Vijay Kumar, Prof Jyoti Chopra, Prof Anand Kumar Srivastava, Prof Parijat Suryavanshi, and Dr Shiv Rajan, all of whom are esteemed faculties and subject experts at King George's Medical University, Lucknow, Uttar Pradesh. We also thank the efforts of our student contributors– Divyansh Ahuja, Divya, and Md. Kaif Khan from King George's Medical University, Lucknow, Uttar Pradesh, and Sanjiban Gupta from North Bengal Medical College, Siliguri, West Bengal.

Dr Anurag Rai would like to thank his parents– Dr AK Rai and Mrs Kusum Rai, and Prof Ravi Kant (Former Vice Chancellor, KGMU) for helping him reach great heights.

Shubhajeet Roy would like to extend his gratitude to his parents– Mr Susanta Roy and Mrs Bratati Roy, grandmother Mrs Kabita Roy, his mentors in KGMU– Prof Archana Ghildiyal (Physiology), Prof Sunita Tiwari (Physiology), Prof Sarvesh Singh (Pharmacology), Prof Abhinav Arun Sonkar (Surgery), Prof Gitika Nanda Singh (Surgery), Prof Harvinder Singh Pahwa (Surgery), Prof Awanish Kumar (Surgery), Prof Ajay Kumar Pal (Surgery), Dr Kushagra Gaurav (Surgery), Prof Sciddhartha Koonwar (Pediatrics), Prof Anand Pandey (Pediatric Surgery), Prof Pooja Ramakant (Endocrine Surgery), Prof Gaurav Chaudhary (Cardiology), Prof Akshyaya Pradhan (Cardiology), Prof Arpit Singh (Orthopedic Surgery), Prof Sujita Kumar Kar (Psychiatry), Dr Jyoti Bajpai (Respiratory Medicine), Dr Harsha Vardhan (Plastic & Reconstructive Surgery), and Dr Sheetal Verma (Microbiology) for their mentorship and helping him achieve great standards in terms of research and academics, his colleagues including Rohit Anand, Suyash Kumar Varshney, Saubhagya Agnihotri, Aditi Shah, Shikhar S Gupta, Shruti Sharma, and Jay Tewari, and juniors like Rachna Singh and Timil Suresh for their unwavering support in times of need and providing moral support.

Mehul Saxena would like to thank his parents Mr Sunil Saxena and Mrs Ritu Saxena, and his elder brother Mr Anshul Saxena for their unconditional support in all his endeavors including this.

The authors are also grateful to the Vice Chancellor of King George's Medical University, Lucknow– Prof Soniya Nityanand, for inspiring young medicos like the authors to take up research and academic works, alongside patient treatment and daily routine duties.

We also acknowledge the efforts put forward by the entire BlueRose Publishers team, who have worked tirelessly towards shaping this book on how it is today.

Contributors

1. **Prof Vijay Kumar,** *MBBS MS (General Surgery) MCh (Surgical Oncology) FICS FACS*

   Professor and Head, Department of Surgical Oncology,

   King George's Medical University, Lucknow

2. **Prof Jyoti Chopra,** *MBBS MS (Anatomy)*

   Professor, Department of Anatomy, and

   Controller of Examinations,

   King George's Medical University, Lucknow

3. **Prof Parijat Suryavanshi,** *MBBS MS (General Surgery) MCh (Surgical Oncology)*

   Professor, Department of Surgery (General),

   King George's Medical University, Lucknow

4. **Prof Anand Kumar Srivastava,** *MBBS MD (Respiratory Medicine)*

   Professor, Department of Respiratory Medicine,

   King George's Medical University, Lucknow

5. **Dr Shiv Rajan,** *MBBS MS (General Surgery) MCh (Surgical Oncology)*

   Associate Professor, Department of Surgical Oncology,

   King George's Medical University, Lucknow

6. **Divyansh Ahuja**

   MBBS Student,

   Faculty of Medical Sciences,

   King George's Medical University, Lucknow

7. **Sanjiban Gupta**

MBBS Student,

North Bengal Medical College, Siliguri

8. **Divya**

MBBS Student,

Faculty of Medical Sciences,

King George's Medical University, Lucknow

9. **Md. Kaif Khan**

MBBS Student,

Faculty of Medical Sciences,

King George's Medical University, Lucknow

Contents

Chapter 1: Chest Wall Anatomy 1

Chapter 2: Chest Wall Physiology 16

Chapter 3: Classification of Chest Wall Tumors 27

Chapter 4: Clinical Presentations and Symptoms 57

Chapter 5: Imaging Techniques, Tissue Biopsy, and Their Role in
    Chest Wall Tumor Diagnosis 66

Chapter 6: Chest-Wall Tumor Management 74

Chapter 7: Multidisciplinary Care and Team Approach 87

Chapter 8: Research and Advancements: 93

Chapter 9: Resource and Support for Patients 100

Chapter 1
Chest Wall Anatomy

Mehul Saxena, Prof Jyoti Chopra

Introduction:

The human chest wall is a remarkable and intricate structure that serves as the protective shield guarding some of our most vital organs. Composed of various skeletal components, intricate vascular networks, and a complex nervous system, the chest wall plays a pivotal role in ensuring our well-being and facilitating the essential functions of respiration. In this chapter, we will embark on a journey to explore the fascinating realm of chest wall anatomy, gaining a profound understanding of its constituent elements and their significance.

The skeletal framework of the chest wall is primarily formed by the ribs and costal cartilages. These skeletal components can be classified into typical and atypical ribs, each with distinct characteristics and roles. The sternum, consisting of three bony parts, anchors the chest wall's central core and plays a crucial role in its functionality. Understanding the anatomy of these skeletal elements is paramount for comprehending chest wall dynamics.

The chest wall is not merely a static structure; it is a dynamic ensemble of muscles that come to life with every breath we take. These chest wall muscles can be categorized into three groups: anterior, posterior, and abdominal muscles. Each group has its unique contribution to respiration and chest wall dynamics, making them integral to our ability to maximize our lung capacity.

Vascular supply to the chest wall is a complex network of arteries and veins, with the internal mammary arteries dominating as the superior blood supply to the sternum. Cutaneous perforators and posterior intercostal arteries also play crucial roles, serving as the foundation for various reconstructive flap procedures and providing essential nourishment to the chest wall and surrounding tissues.

The nervous system of the chest wall is intricately woven with intercostal nerves, which contribute to muscle contraction and sensory feedback from the skin and pleura. These nerves emerge from the thoracic spinal nerves and ensure the proper functioning of the chest wall. The classification of intercostal nerves into typical and atypical categories underscores their unique roles and pathways within the human body.

The significance of understanding chest wall anatomy extends beyond the realms of medical knowledge. This knowledge is vital for protective functions, surgical considerations, and clinical implications. The chest wall serves as a protective enclosure around our vital organs, and disruptions in its structure can lead to severe respiratory and circulatory issues. For surgeons and medical practitioners, knowledge of chest wall anatomy is crucial for safe and successful procedures. Additionally, the clinical significance of chest wall anatomy is evident in conditions like intercostal neuralgia, where precision in treatment is essential.

Skeletal Components:

Ribs

The chest wall's lateral framework is primarily formed by the ribs and costal cartilages. Ribs can be categorised into two main groups: typical and atypical.

1. Typical Ribs

Typical ribs (Ribs 3-10) attach to the spinal column posteriorly and connect to the sternum by costal cartilages anteriorly. They consist of a head, neck, tubercle, articular facet, and shaft. Typical ribs articulate with the costal cartilages through a frontal cup. A notable feature is the presence of a notch on the underside, housing essential structures such as the intercostal nerve, artery, and vein.

2. Atypical Ribs

Among the atypical ribs, Ribs 1-2 and Ribs 11-12 have distinct characteristics and limited mobility. Rib 1 is flat and has a single facet on its head, contributing minimally to chest wall expansion. Rib 2 is relatively larger but less prominent than typical ribs and may have a less defined costal groove.

Floating Ribs

Ribs 11 and 12, known as floating ribs, possess single facets on their heads and rudimentary cartilages. These ribs do not connect with the rest of the rib cage and are aptly named for their floating quality.

Sternum

The sternum, consisting of three bony parts connected by two joints, is a central component of the chest wall. Understanding its anatomy is crucial for comprehending chest wall functionality.

Manubrium

At the cephalad end of the sternum is the large, flat, wide manubrium. It primarily articulates with the first rib and the clavicle, offering limited anterior and upward movement. The first and second ribs, relatively short and flat, contribute minimally to the increase in the chest's internal diameter.

Gladiolus

The gladiolus, the largest and flattest part of the sternum, articulates with Ribs 2 through 7. Rib 7 joins the sternum at the junction between the xiphoid process and the gladiolus. The movement of the gladiolus, when the sternum is in motion, draws the attached ribs upward and outward, significantly increasing the chest's transverse diameter.

Xiphoid Process

The xiphoid process, though small, is the inferior-most part of the sternum. While it partially articulates with the seventh rib, it has limited significance in chest wall anatomy and physiology.

Costal Cartilage

Costal cartilages are integral to the articulation of the ribs with the sternum anteriorly. These cartilages facilitate coordinated movement during respiration.

Articulation with the Sternum

Costal cartilages 1 through 7 directly articulate with the sternum. Cartilages 7 and 8 often fuse at their margins where they connect to the sternum. Ribs 8, 9, and 10 combine to form the costal arch, which also connects with the sternum. Ribs 1 and 2 have relatively small cartilages, offering limited movement.

Joints:

The joints within the chest wall can be categorised based on their location as either anterior or posterior. While anterior joints mainly involve the sternum and costal cartilages, posterior joints, which are more intricate, encompass the interaction between ribs and the vertebral column.

Posterior Joints

Posterior joints, characterized by their complexity, involve the articulation of ribs with two vertebral bodies and one transverse process. In general, typical or common ribs possess two facets each for articulation. The upper facet connects with the vertebral body above the rib, while the lower facet on the rib's head articulates with the vertebral body below the rib.

The tubercle of the rib engages with the transverse processes of the corresponding vertebral body, forming a crucial connection point often likened to a 'bucket handle' joining a 'bucket.' This posterior articulation enables the rib to swing upward, while the anterior articulations play a pivotal role in elevating the rib, bringing it and associated structures cephalad, and increasing the interthoracic diameter of the chest.

Anterior Joints

Anterior joints involve the connection between the sternum and the ribs laterally, facilitated by the intervening costal cartilages. These cartilages directly articulate with their respective ribs and subsequently move anteriorly. Along the lower four ribs, they fuse as they approach the sternum.

The sternum, acting as a central anchor, elevates the entire arch of ribs as a cohesive unit, drawing all the ribs' arches anteriorly and cephalad. This orchestrated movement increases the internal diameter of the chest, a crucial element in various physiological processes.

Musculature

The musculature of the chest wall, diverse in its location and anatomy, is fundamental to respiration and maximizing its capacity to its fullest [1]. These muscles can be categorized into three groups based on their anatomical locations.

Anterior Chest Wall Muscles

Located at the anterior aspect of the chest, these muscles are vital for chest wall dynamics and include the:

Pectoralis Major Muscle

The pectoralis major muscle, a fan-shaped structure covering the anterior superior chest, attaches proximally to the clavicle, sternum, and costal cartilages and distally to the humerus. Its primary blood supply is from the thoracoacromial artery, supplemented by segmental branches from the internal mammary artery [3]. This versatile muscle can be raised as a muscle or musculocutaneous flap and is employed in various flap-based reconstruction techniques. It plays a pivotal role in closing central anterior chest defects [2].

Posterior Chest Wall Muscles

Situated at the posterior aspect of the chest, these muscles contribute significantly to chest wall movements and include the:

Serratus Anterior Muscle

The serratus anterior muscle, classified as a type II muscle flap, receives its blood supply from the lateral thoracic artery and branches of the subscapular thoracodorsal artery [2]. The arterial branches contribute to the complex vascular network of this muscle, providing versatility in its use for flap-based reconstruction [4, 5]. The serratus anterior muscle, with its role in shoulder movement and its excellent vascular pedicle, becomes a valuable option for addressing intrathoracic defects and composite chest wall reconstructions [6, 7].

Abdominal Muscles

The abdominal muscles, though not exclusively chest wall muscles, are integral in chest wall dynamics and include the:

Rectus Abdominis, Internal Oblique, and External Oblique Muscles

These muscles are involved in decreasing lung volumes by constricting the rib cage in a downward motion during exhalation. They also contribute to pushing the viscera cephalad, thereby elevating the diaphragm and aiding in the exhalation process [1].

In conclusion, the chest wall's musculature comprises a diverse array of muscles, each with its unique location and anatomy [1].

Vasculature

Superior Blood Supply to the Sternum

Internal Mammary Arteries

The dominant blood supply to the sternum is primarily provided superiorly by the paired internal mammary (or thoracic) arteries. These arteries originate as branches of the subclavian artery and course behind the costal cartilages, running alongside the sternum. They interconnect with other critical vessels, including the posterior intercostals, lateral thoracic, acromio-thoracic, and transverse cervical arteries [2]. Often accompanied by one or two venae comitantes, these arteries play a pivotal role in the vascularization of the chest wall. Additionally, ventral skin and musculature receive their superior blood supply through collateralization of branches of the subclavian vessels, extending inferiorly to the deep epigastric arteries. This interconnected vascular system serves as the foundation for various reconstructive flap procedures [2].

Cutaneous Perforators

Around the perimeter of the pectoralis major muscle, along the costal margin, and within the interdigitations of the serratus anterior muscle in the midaxillary line, cutaneous perforators of these vessels are concentrated. These perforators are of significant importance in the context of vascular supply to the chest wall [8].

Predominant Blood Supply to the Breast

In clinical studies, Marcus noted that the internal mammary artery predominately supplies blood to the breast in 68 to 74% of patients, with its dominance surpassing that of the lateral thoracic artery [9]. Remarkably, the largest internal mammary artery perforators, consistently located in the second or third intercostal space, are integral to the blood supply of the internal mammary artery perforator flap [10-12].

Intercostal Vessels

Within each intercostal space, the intercostal vessels travel in close association with the intercostal nerves. These vessels include the anterior and posterior intercostal arteries, both playing a pivotal role in chest wall vascular supply.

Posterior Intercostal Arteries

The largest angiosome in the torso is primarily supplied by the posterior intercostal arteries [13]. Kerrigan and Daniel have extensively described cutaneous flaps based on the intercostal arteries, outlining the course of the intercostal neurovascular bundle. This bundle is divided into four segments: vertebral, costal groove, intermuscular, and rectus [2]. Dorsal perforators of the posterior intercostal arteries, branching from the vertebral segment, with an average diameter of 1.5 mm, serve as the foundation for the dorsal intercostal artery perforator flap [15].

Anterior Intercostal Arteries

The anterior intercostal arteries, originating as branches of the internal thoracic artery, provide blood supply to the upper six intercostal spaces. Beyond this point, the internal thoracic artery terminates by dividing into the superior epigastric artery and musculophrenic artery [26]. The musculophrenic artery subsequently supplies the remaining anterior intercostal branches, which then anastomose with the posterior intercostal arteries arising from the thoracic aorta [26]. Notably, the right posterior intercostal arteries are longer than their left counterparts due to the aorta's leftward position relative to the vertebral column [18].

Each posterior intercostal artery runs along the lower border of the corresponding rib, accompanied by a posterior intercostal vein and intercostal nerve. Throughout most of their course, the intercostal nerve lies inferior to the intercostal artery, while the intercostal vein lies superior to the artery [19].

Understanding this intricate vascular network is essential for surgical procedures, particularly reconstructive flaps, and significantly contributes to the chest wall's functional dynamics.

Nervous System of the Chest Wall

The intercostal nerves play a pivotal role within the somatic nervous system, contributing to muscle contraction and sensory information retrieval from the skin and parietal pleura. These nerves emerge from the anterior rami of the thoracic spinal nerves spanning from T1 to T11. Positioned neatly between adjacent ribs, they ensure the proper functioning of the chest wall [26].

Anatomical Distinctions

The twelfth thoracic nerve's anterior division, while closely related, is technically not classified as an intercostal nerve. Instead, it is referred to as the subcostal nerve, as it descends below the ribs to enter the abdominal wall, serving distinct functions [26]. These nerves are vital not only for motor function but also in the context of analgesia and pathology, with certain techniques involving nerve blockage and potential neuralgia-related issues [26].

Structure and Pathway

Each intercostal nerve enters the corresponding intercostal space, situated between the posterior intercostal membrane and the parietal pleura [26]. It then proceeds to descend into the subcostal groove of the associated rib, located directly inferior to the rib [26]. Along this course, the nerve finds itself bordered by the innermost intercostal muscle and the internal intercostal muscle [26]. Notably, the first six intercostal nerves extend branches and culminate within their respective intercostal spaces, just below the corresponding rib. In contrast, the seventh through eleventh intercostal nerves deviate from the intercostal spaces and venture into the abdominal wall. This unique path classifies them as thoracoabdominal nerves [16,17].

Classification of Intercostal Nerves

The intercostal nerves can be categorized into two distinct groups: typical intercostal nerves and atypical intercostal nerves. The differentiation arises from the spatial confinement of the typical intercostal nerves within their respective intercostal spaces, whereas atypical spinal nerves traverse beyond the confines of the thoracic wall to partially or entirely serve other regions [20].

Typical Intercostal Nerves (IC3 through IC6)

Typical intercostal nerves exhibit a characteristic course, traveling laterally behind the sympathetic trunk before entering the intercostal space between the parietal pleura and the intercostal membrane [26]. Within the costal groove, they share space with the intercostal vessels and traverse anterior to the internal thoracic artery. Notably, these nerves give rise to several crucial branches, including the rami communicantes, muscular branches, collateral branch, lateral cutaneous branch, and anterior cutaneous branch [26].

- The rami communicantes facilitate visceral signaling to and from the corresponding thoracic ganglion via gray and white rami.

- Muscular branches supply the intercostal muscles, along with the serratus posterior superior, subcostal, transversus thoracis, and levatores costarum.

- The collateral branch provides innervation to the intercostal muscles, parietal pleura, and rib periosteum.

- The lateral cutaneous branch traverses the lateral thoracic wall muscles and subsequently divides into anterior and posterior branches, responsible for sensory feedback from the skin in the lateral thoracic wall.

- The anterior cutaneous branch, representing the terminal branch, further divides into medial and lateral branches, supplying sensory innervation to the anterior thoracic wall [21].

Atypical Intercostal Nerves (IC1, IC2, IC8 through IC11)

Atypical intercostal nerves, including IC1 through IC2 and IC8 through IC11, embark on more intricate journeys, each possessing unique routes to innervation within the human body.

- The first intercostal nerve contributes, albeit to a limited extent, to the lower trunk of the brachial plexus, alongside the anterior ramus of C8. Notably, it lacks both lateral and anterior cutaneous branches found in typical intercostal nerves.

- The second intercostal nerve features a branch known as the intercostobrachial nerve, responsible for sensory feedback from the floor of the axilla and the superior region of the upper extremity. In cases of coronary artery disease, this nerve can elicit the cardiac pain experienced on the medial side of the arm.

- The seventh to eleventh intercostal nerves, while initially traversing intercostal spaces, ultimately diverge into the abdominal wall. Here, they supply muscles such as the external oblique, internal oblique, transversus abdominis, and rectus abdominis, as well as innervate the skin and parietal peritoneum [22].

Importance of Chest Wall Anatomy

Protective Function

- The chest wall acts as a protective enclosure around vital organs.
- Disruption in its structure can lead to severe respiratory and circulatory issues.
- Advancements in managing complex chest wall defects include using muscle and musculocutaneous flaps.
- Flaps like latissimus dorsi, pectoralis major, serratus anterior, and rectus abdominis have reduced infections and mortality.
- Successful reconstruction relies on understanding chest wall anatomy and its role in specific diseases [2].

Surgical Considerations

- Intercostal nerves are at risk during thoracotomies and chest tube placements.

- Safe chest tube placement involves careful intercostal space dissection.

- Anesthetic blocks of intercostal nerves before thoracotomy closure may affect blood pressure [23,24] [26].

Clinical Significance

- Intercostal neuralgia is common, causing sharp, burning, or shooting pain.

- Pain typically starts at the posterior axillary line and radiates anteriorly.

- Pain worsens with deep breaths, affecting breathing patterns.

- Treatment options include medications (antidepressants, anticonvulsants), non-somatic treatments, and nerve blocks.

- Nerve blocks require precise technique due to their proximity to the pleural space [25] [26].

References:

1. Graeber GM, Nazim M. The anatomy of the ribs and the sternum and their relationship to chest wall structure and function. Thoracic surgery clinics. 2007 Nov 1;17(4):473-89.

2. Clemens MW, Evans KK, Mardini S, Arnold PG. Introduction to chest wall reconstruction: anatomy and physiology of the chest and indications for chest wall reconstruction. InSeminars in plastic surgery 2011 Feb (Vol. 25, No. 01, pp. 005-015). © Thieme Medical Publishers.

3. Nahai F, Morales Jr L, Bone DK, Bostwick III J. Pectoralis major muscle turnover flaps for closure of the infected sternotomy

wound with preservation of form and function. Plastic and Reconstructive Surgery. 1982 Oct 1;70(4):471-4.

4. Mathes SJ, Nahai F, Friedman VM. Clinical atlas of muscle and musculocutaneous flaps. St. Louis: Mosby; 1979 Jan.

5. Bartlett SP, May Jr JW, Yaremchuk MJ. The latissimus dorsi muscle: a fresh cadaver study of the primary neurovascular pedicle. Plastic and reconstructive surgery. 1981 May 1;67(5):631-6.

6. Arnold PG, Pairolero PC, Waldorf JC. The serratus anterior muscle: intrathoracic and extrathoracic utilization. Plastic and reconstructive surgery. 1984 Feb 1;73(2):240-6.

7. Inoue T, Ohba S, Takamatus A, Kitazawa T, Harashina T. Chest wall reconstruction using pedicled extended serratus anterior myocutaneous flap combined with vascularized rib. European Journal of Plastic Surgery. 1996 Mar;19:97-9.

8. Palmer JH, Taylor GI. The vascular territories of the anterior chest wall. British journal of plastic surgery. 1986 Jul 1;39(3):287-99.

9. Marcus GH. Untersuchungen uber die arterielle Blutversorgung der Mamilla. Arch Klin Chir. 1934;179:361-9.

10. Rosson GD, Holton LH, Silverman RP, Singh NK, Nahabedian MY. Internal mammary perforators: a cadaver study. Journal of reconstructive microsurgery. 2005 May;21(04):239-42.

11. Neligan PC, Gullane PJ, Vesely M, Murray D. The internal mammary artery perforator flap: New variation on an old theme. Plastic and reconstructive surgery. 2007 Mar 1;119(3):891-3.

12. Wong C, Saint-Cyr M, Rasko Y, Mojallal A, Bailey S, Myers S, Rohrich RJ. Three-and four-dimensional arterial and venous perforasomes of the internal mammary artery perforator flap. Plastic and reconstructive surgery. 2009 Dec 1;124(6):1759-69.

13. Taylor GI, Minabe T. The angiosomes of the mammals and other vertebrates. Plastic and reconstructive surgery. 1992 Feb 1;89(2):181-215.

14. Kerrigan CL, Daniel RK. The intercostal flap: an anatomical and hemodynamic approach. Annals of Plastic Surgery. 1979 May 1;2(5):411-21.

15. Minabe T, Harii K. Dorsal intercostal artery perforator flap: anatomical study and clinical applications. Plastic and reconstructive surgery. 2007 Sep 1;120(3):681-9.

16. Mayes J, Davison E, Panahi P, Patten D, Eljelani F, Womack J, Varma M. An anatomical evaluation of the serratus anterior plane block. Anaesthesia. 2016 Sep;71(9):1064-9.

17. Kommuru H, Jothi S, Bapuji P, Antony J. Thoracic part of sympathetic chain and its branching pattern variations in South Indian cadavers. Journal of Clinical and Diagnostic Research: JCDR. 2014 Dec;8(12):AC09.

18. Iida T, Narushima M, Yoshimatsu H, Mihara M, Kikuchi K, Hara H, Yamamoto T, Araki J, Koshima I. Versatility of lateral cutaneous branches of intercostal vessels and nerves: anatomical study and clinical application. Journal of Plastic, Reconstructive & Aesthetic Surgery. 2013 Nov 1;66(11):1564-8.

19. Palussière J, Canella M, Cornelis F, Catena V, Descat E, Brouste V, Montaudon M. Retrospective review of thoracic neural damage during lung ablation–what the interventional radiologist needs to know about neural thoracic anatomy. Cardiovascular and interventional radiology. 2013 Dec;36:1602-13.

20. Haam S, Kim D, Hwang J, Paik H, Lee D. An anatomical study of the relationship between the sympathetic trunk and intercostal veins of the third and fourth intercostal spaces during thoracoscopy. Clinical Anatomy. 2010 Sep;23(6):702-6.

21. Miyawaki M. Constancy and characteristics of the anterior cutaneous branch of the first intercostal nerve: correcting the

descriptions in human anatomy texts. Anatomical science international. 2006 Dec;81:225-41.

22. Wraight WM, Tweedie DJ, Parkin IG. Neurovascular anatomy and variation in the fourth, fifth, and sixth intercostal spaces in the mid-axillary line: a cadaveric study in respect of chest drain insertion. Clinical Anatomy: The Official Journal of the American Association of Clinical Anatomists and the British Association of Clinical Anatomists. 2005 Jul;18(5):346-9.

23. Ueshima H, Hara E, Marui T, Otake H. RETRACTED: The ultrasound-guided transversus thoracic muscle plane block is effective for the median sternotomy. Journal of Clinical Anesthesia. 2016 Feb 9;29:83-.

24. Fujii S, Vissa D, Ganapathy S, Johnson M, Zhou J. Transversus thoracic muscle plane block on a cadaver with history of coronary artery bypass grafting. Regional Anesthesia and Pain Medicine. 2017 Jul 1;42(4):535-7.

25. Jammes Y, Delpierre S. Respiratory and circulatory effects of parietal pleural afferent stimulation in rabbits. Journal of Applied Physiology. 2006 May;100(5):1539-46.

26. Glenesk NL, Rahman S, Lopez PP. Anatomy, thorax, intercostal nerves.

Chapter 2
Chest Wall Physiology

Divyansh Ahuja, Prof Anand Kumar Srivastava

Introduction

The inspiratory and expiratory muscles of the rib cage work in a precisely coordinated movement to execute a functional breath. In the pleural cavity, the lung remains inflated by mechanical coupling of the chest wall and the lung[1]. The work of breathing is minimized by mesothelial cells with microvilli that are enmeshed in hyaluronic acid–rich lubricants [2]. Elevated movement of the ribs leads to forced inspiration by increasing the dimensions of the chest through a "bucket-handle" motion and by elevation of the sternum through a "pump-handle" motion.

The muscles of inspiration work actively to create a reduced intrapleural pressure to induce inhalation [3]. Because of its distinctive curved geometry and specialized metabolic demands, the diaphragm is the most important respiratory muscle [4]. With assistance from the external intercostal muscles, the diaphragm contracts during inspiration to enlarge the thoracic cavity. Paired sternocleidomastoids and scalene muscles act as secondary accessory muscles to aid in raising the sternum and elevating the upper ribs [1].

Mechanism of respiration

For understanding the mechanics of respiration in a simplified manner, a straightforward analogy involves likening it to a cylinder with a piston [5]. The ribs, costal cartilages, and sternum collectively provide a sturdy framework for the cylindrical structure, while the diaphragm serves as the piston [5]. During calm and resting breathing, the diaphragm contracts, lowering the central tendon and generating a negative pressure within the chest [5]. This occurs because the ribs, costal cartilages, and sternum maintain the chest wall's fixed cylindrical form. The lungs, intimately connected to the chest wall through pleural surfaces, respond by expanding as they follow the created negative intrathoracic pressure [5]. Following the completion of inhalation, the diaphragm relaxes, and the inherent elastic nature of the lungs prompts them to contract toward their original volume, instigating exhalation. In quiet respiration, the chest wall experiences minimal to no movement [5].

Role of diaphragm in breathing

The diaphragm is the primary respiratory muscle in the human body, responsible for approximately 80% of the work involved in normal tidal breathing [24]. While the process of breathing may seem involuntary, the effective functioning and mechanical efficiency of the diaphragm depend significantly on its anatomical arrangement in relation to the lower rib cage. The region where the diaphragm attaches to the rib cage is known as the Zone of Apposition (ZOA). It extends from the diaphragm's caudal insertion near the costal margin and moves cephalad to the costophrenic angle, where the muscle fibers disengage from the rib cage to form the free diaphragmatic dome [24]. The ZOA plays a pivotal role in maintaining efficient length-tension relationships within the diaphragm. This includes keeping the vertical alignment of diaphragmatic muscle fibers and enabling postero-lateral (bucket-handle) movement of the lower rib cage. During quiet inhalation, the diaphragm contracts, causing a reduction in its axial length and a descent of the diaphragmatic dome concerning its costal insertions [6,7].

In the inhalation phase of ventilation, as the diaphragm contracts and moves towards the abdominal cavity, intra-abdominal pressure increases. This action results in the three-dimensional distension of the abdominal wall, accompanied by an outward rotation of the ribs. The abdominal wall opposes the diaphragm's action through an eccentric contraction involving all abdominal muscles. This eccentric contraction is crucial in controlling the length-tension relationship of the diaphragmatic muscle [24]. It helps maintain the dome shape of the diaphragm and prolongs the Zone of Apposition, thereby facilitating the postero-lateral expansion of the lower rib cage and enhancing the force generated by the diaphragm. Furthermore, reduced activity of the abdominal muscles permits visceral displacement due to the diaphragmatic dome's descent. This action is reversed during expiration [5].

Role of intercostal muscles

Amberger proposed a classification of intercostal muscles, designating the external intercostals as inspiratory muscles and the internal intercostals as expiratory muscles, except for the intercartilaginous portion, which plays an inspiratory role [8].

When an intercostal muscle contracts within a specific interspace, it exerts a downward force on the upper rib and an upward force on the lower rib. However, due to the orientation of the fibers in the external intercostal muscles, which slope caudally and ventrally from the rib above to the rib below, their lower insertion point is situated farther from the central pivot point of rib rotation (i.e., the costovertebral articulations) than their upper insertion [9]. Consequently, when these fibers contract and apply equal and opposing forces at both insertions, the torque exerted on the lower rib, which tends to elevate it, surpasses the torque on the upper rib, which tends to depress it. Therefore, the primary effect of the external intercostal muscles is to elevate the ribs, resulting in lung inflation [9].

Conversely, the fibers of the internal intercostal muscles slope caudally and dorsally from the rib above to the rib below, such that their lower insertion is closer to the central pivot point of rib rotation than their upper insertion [9]. This configuration results in a smaller torque on the lower rib compared to the upper rib when the muscle contracts. Consequently, the net effect of the internal intercostal muscles is to depress the ribs, leading to lung deflation [9].

Chest wall compliance and elasticity

Compliance within the respiratory system pertains to the expansibility of both the lungs and the chest wall. It is categorized into two distinct types: dynamic and static compliance. Dynamic compliance is a measure of compliance taken during the act of breathing, encompassing a composite of lung compliance and airway resistance [10]. Conversely, to gauge static compliance, it is imperative to assess the volume variations resulting from alterations in the driving pressure applied across the respiratory system [11].

Furthermore, the compliance of the respiratory system depends on two critical factors: the elastic recoil of the lungs and the surface tension exerted by the fluid present within the alveoli.

In the realm of intensive care, compliance measurements assume considerable importance and utility. They are routinely evaluated in patients afflicted with conditions characterized by stiffened lungs, such as individuals suffering from acute respiratory distress syndrome (ARDS), who necessitate mechanical ventilation [11].

Elasticity of lungs

The mechanical characteristics of lung tissue play a substantial role in shaping the physiological functions and overall behavior of the respiratory system. These characteristics are intricately linked to both elastic and resistive forces [12].

Surfactant of lung and its effect on surface tension

Human lung surfactant is a complex mixture comprising lipids and proteins, which forms a monolayer at the interface between alveolar liquid and air. Of the phospholipids present, 80% consist of phosphatidylcholine, while 9% are phosphatidylglycerol. Among the phosphatidylcholines, over half (55%) are saturated and contain more than 70% palmitic acid. In contrast, phosphatidylglycerol contains 22% palmitic acid and 52% oleic acid, suggesting that the significance of phosphatidylglycerol in surfactant function is linked to its acidic head group. Human surfactant primarily consists of high molecular weight glycoproteins [13], and it is secreted by specialized surfactant-secreting epithelial cells known as type 2 epithelial cells [14].

Age related changes

Total respiratory system compliance encompasses both lung and chest wall compliance, representing the change in volume relative to changes in pressure. Lung compliance influences the speed and force of expiration, while thoracic compliance is responsible for managing the elastic load during inhalation. As individuals age, structural alterations in the thoracic cage occur, leading to a reduction in chest wall compliance [15] along with that there is increased stiffness in the parenchyma regions of the lung however this might seem counterintuitive because numerous studies have indicated that the lungs and the respiratory system tend to become more compliant as individuals age [15,16]. Also, aging has a significant impact on the mechanical properties of both blood vessels and parenchymal tissue, with the vascular compartment experiencing the most substantial rate of change [17]. The natural aging process is associated with molecular and physiological modifications that result in shifts in lung function, reduced pulmonary remodeling and regenerative capacity, and heightened susceptibility to acute and chronic lung ailments [19]. Furthermore, exposure to extrinsic factors related to the passage of time, such as chronic exposure to atmospheric pollution, dust, particulates, and gases, can inflict minor insults on cellular function and accelerate lung aging [18]. While the number of alveoli, alveolar ducts, and capillary segments remains relatively constant in adulthood, there is a noticeable increase in alveolar size and alveolar-capillary surface area with aging [20]. A decline in elastic recoil, coupled with a decrease in the number of elastic attachments supporting alveoli and an increase in collagen, leads to the closure of smaller airways at higher lung volumes. Consequently, in older individuals, some airways may become narrowed or closed during regular tidal breathing, resulting in an increase in functional residual capacity and a reduction in expiratory airflow from the lungs [19]. All the above-mentioned changes lead to decreased pulmonary functioning.

Cellular changes in aged lung

Cellular alterations in the aging lung play a significant role in respiratory health. The respiratory airway's epithelial surface is a critical area for efficient gas exchange and host defense, relying heavily on the integrity of the epithelium. Age-related changes in the composition and functioning of type 1 and type 2 epithelial cells, airway smooth muscle cells, and fibroblasts can contribute to the development and progression of lung disorders in the elderly. Furthermore, poor prognosis and recovery in pulmonary inflammatory diseases are often linked to immunosenescence, which involves age-related changes in the innate and adaptive immune responses in the lung [19].

Immunological changes

Innate Immunity:

There is a decline in phagocytic capacity in alveolar and pulmonary macrophages associated with aging, resulting in impaired or delayed pathogen clearance from the lung [21].

Age-related alterations in pathogen recognition, reduced expression of pattern recognition receptors (PRRs), and decreased responses to secondary signaling pathways may contribute to the increased susceptibility of older individuals to infectious agents [22].

Dendritic cells, crucial orchestrators of the immune response, play a key role in immunity generation and tolerance maintenance. However, their functions are compromised with age. While the numbers and phenotype of dendritic cell subsets in aged individuals are not significantly affected, their ability to phagocytose antigens and migrate is impaired [23].

Adaptive Immunity:

In the T-cell mediated adaptive immune response, multiple age-related changes in T-cell numbers and function are associated with increased susceptibility of older individuals to environmental stimuli. The populations of CD3+, CD4+, and CD8+ T cells decrease with age [19].

Memory T-cell responses, diversity in the T-cell receptor repertoire, differentiation of T-helper cells, and T-helper cell activity all decline with age [24,25].

B-cell mediated:

Immature B-cell migration is affected, and there is an increase in age-associated B cells, leading to decreased repertoire diversity [26].

Although the functional ability to produce antibodies remains intact, age-related changes in antibody specificity and antigen affinity result in a reduced capacity to generate large antibody responses in older individuals [26].

Assessment of chest wall function

Spirometry is a valuable diagnostic tool used to measure the volume of air (in liters) exhaled or inhaled by patients over time. It serves as a powerful means of detecting, monitoring, and managing individuals with lung disorders. Indications for performing spirometry include persistent cough, exposure to lung irritants, chest pain, and the use of potentially lung-toxic medications [29].

In primary care settings, spirometry is particularly useful for diagnosing obstructive lung diseases, which are prevalent. There are simplified algorithms that can aid in distinguishing obstructive conditions from other respiratory issues based solely on spirometry results [28].

Regarding incentive spirometry, its clinical effectiveness remains a topic of debate, even though it is commonly employed in perioperative respiratory therapy as part of routine preventive and therapeutic protocols [27].

To assess chest wall motion, various physical devices like magnetometers or accelerometers have been used to measure increases in the anterior-posterior (AP) diameter. Other techniques, such as respiratory inductive plethysmography (RIP) and structured-light plethysmography, have also been employed [30]. Many of these methods for evaluating chest wall motion can yield indicators of tidal expiratory airflow patterns and thoracoabdominal asynchrony, which indirectly serve as markers of respiratory disease [31].

In the realm of radiological techniques, magnetic resonance imaging (MRI) has been applied to examine detailed aspects of chest wall motion in adults or adolescents. This examination can occur during breath-holding, deep breathing, or tidal breathing [31].

References

1. Clemens MW, Evans KK, Mardini S, Arnold PG. Introduction to chest wall reconstruction: anatomy and physiology of the chest and indications for chest wall reconstruction. InSeminars in plastic surgery 2011 Feb (Vol. 25, No. 01, pp. 005-015). © Thieme Medical Publishers.

2. Wang NS. Anatomy and physiology of the pleural space. Clinics in chest medicine. 1985 Mar 1;6(1):3-16.

3. Fell GE. Forced respiration. Medical Record (1866-1922). 1890 Feb 22;37(8):225.

4. Goldman MD, Mead JE. Mechanical interaction between the diaphragm and rib cage. Journal of Applied Physiology. 1973 Aug;35(2):197-204.

5. Graeber GM, Nazim M. The anatomy of the ribs and the sternum and their relationship to chest wall structure and function. Thoracic surgery clinics. 2007 Nov 1;17(4):473-89.

6. Goldman MD, Mead JE. Mechanical interaction between the diaphragm and rib cage. Journal of Applied Physiology. 1973 Aug;35(2):197-204.

7. Mead J. Functional significance of the area of apposition of diaphragm to rib cage. American Review of Respiratory Disease. 1979 Feb;119(2P2):31-2.

8. Hamberger GE. De respirationis mechanismo et usu genuino diss.(etc.). Croeker; 1749.

9. De Troyer A, Kirkwood PA, Wilson TA. Respiratory action of the intercostal muscles. Physiological reviews. 2005 Apr;85(2):717-56.

10. Edwards Z, Annamaraju P. Physiology, lung compliance. InStatPearls [Internet] 2022 Mar 18. StatPearls Publishing.

11. Kraman S. Lesser used tests of pulmonary function: compliance, resistance and dead space. COPD: Journal of Chronic Obstructive Pulmonary Disease. 2007 Jan 1;4(1):49-54.

12. Bates JH. Lung mechanics: an inverse modeling approach. Cambridge University Press; 2009 Jul 30.

13. Shelley SA, Balis JU, Paciga JE, Espinoza CG, Richman AV. Biochemical composition of adult human lung surfactant. Lung. 1982 Dec;160:195-206.

14. Zuo YY, Veldhuizen RA, Neumann AW, Petersen NO, Possmayer F. Current perspectives in pulmonary surfactant—inhibition, enhancement and evaluation. Biochimica et Biophysica Acta (BBA)-Biomembranes. 2008 Oct 1;1778(10):1947-77.

15. Sharma G, Goodwin J. Effect of aging on respiratory system physiology and immunology. Clinical interventions in aging. 2006 Jan 1;1(3):253-60.

16. Janssens JP, Pache JC, Nicod LP. Physiological changes in respiratory function associated with ageing. European Respiratory Journal. 1999 Jan 1;13(1):197-205.

17. Sicard D, Haak AJ, Choi KM, Craig AR, Fredenburgh LE, Tschumperlin DJ. Aging and anatomical variations in lung tissue stiffness. American Journal of Physiology-Lung Cellular and Molecular Physiology. 2018 Jun 1;314(6):L946-55.

18. Childs BG, Durik M, Baker DJ, Van Deursen JM. Cellular senescence in aging and age-related disease: from mechanisms to therapy. Nature medicine. 2015 Dec;21(12):1424-35.

19. Cho SJ, Stout-Delgado HW. Aging and lung disease. Annual review of physiology. 2020 Feb 10;82:433-59.

20. Quirk JD, Sukstanskii AL, Woods JC, Lutey BA, Conradi MS, Gierada DS, Yusen RD, Castro M, Yablonskiy DA. Experimental evidence of age-related adaptive changes in human acinar airways. Journal of Applied Physiology. 2016 Jan 15;120(2):159-65.

21. Wong CK, Smith CA, Sakamoto K, Kaminski N, Koff JL, Goldstein DR. Aging impairs alveolar macrophage phagocytosis and increases influenza-induced mortality in mice. The Journal of Immunology. 2017 Aug 1;199(3):1060-8.

22. Shaw AC, Panda A, Joshi SR, Qian F, Allore HG, Montgomery RR. Dysregulation of human Toll-like receptor function in aging. Ageing research reviews. 2011 Jul 1;10(3):346-53.

23. Agrawal A, Gupta S. Impact of aging on dendritic cell functions in humans. Ageing research reviews. 2011 Jul 1;10(3):336-45.

24. Kocjan J, Adamek M, Gzik-Zroska B, Czyżewski D, Rydel M. Network of breathing. Multifunctional role of the diaphragm: a

review. Advances in respiratory medicine. 2017 Sep;85(4):224-32.

25. Kovaiou RD, Grubeck-Loebenstein B. Age-associated changes within CD4+ T cells. Immunology letters. 2006 Sep 15;107(1):8-14.

26. Haynes L, Swain SL. Why aging T cells fail: implications for vaccination. Immunity. 2006 Jun 1;24(6):663-6.

27. Holodick NE, Rothstein TL. B cells in the aging immune system: time to consider B-1 cells. Annals of the New York Academy of Sciences. 2015 Dec;1362(1):176-87.

28. Rosière J, Grant K, Larcinese A, Revelly JP, Fittin JW, Sokol C. Appropriateness of respiratory care: evidence-based guidelines. Swiss Medical Weekly. 2009 Jul 11;139(2728):387-.

29. Pellegrino R, Viegi G, Brusasco V, Crapo RO, Burgos F, Casaburi RE, Coates A, Van Der Grinten CP, Gustafsson P, Hankinson J, Jensen R. Interpretative strategies for lung function tests. European respiratory journal. 2005 Nov 1;26(5):948-68.

30. Petty TL, Weinmann GG. Building a national strategy for the prevention and management of and research in chronic obstructive pulmonary disease: National Heart, Lung, and Blood Institute workshop summary. Jama. 1997 Jan 15;277(3):246-53.

31. Tukanova K, Papi E, Jamel S, Hanna GB, McGregor AH, Markar SR. Assessment of chest wall movement following thoracotomy: a systematic review. Journal of Thoracic Disease. 2020 Mar;12(3):1031.

32. Seddon P. Options for assessing and measuring chest wall motion. Paediatric Respiratory Reviews. 2015 Jan 1;16(1):3-10.

Chapter 3
Classification of Chest Wall Tumors

Sanjiban Gupta, Prof Parijat Suryavanshi

Introduction:

The structures surrounding and protecting the lungs, contained by the spine and divided from the abdomen by the diaphragm, are referred to as the chest wall. A variety of tissues are included in these structures, including cartilage, bone, muscle, fascia, vasculature, lymphatic vessels, fat, and skin. Tumors of the chest wall are classified into two types: main and secondary. Primary chest wall tumors develop from the chest wall's muscle, fat, blood vessels, nerve sheath, cartilage, or bone. Secondary chest wall cancers can occur as a result of direct invasion of breast or lung carcinoma or as metastases from a distant site of origin. On the surface, chest wall tumors can be difficult to identify; nevertheless, a thorough history and physical examination can lead to proper imaging and management. It is critical to study the various imaging modalities available and what information may be obtained by ordering the appropriate modality. A biopsy is the gold standard for making a definitive diagnosis, and surgical options can be considered with the patient, with the necessary risks and benefits addressed. Because these chest wall tumors affect a wide range of specializations and providers, it is critical to adopt an interprofessional approach to patient treatment.

Chest wall tumors are caused by benign or malignant cellular expansion and proliferation, as well as infectious or inflammatory events.

Tumors of the bone, muscle, fat, blood vessels, nerve sheaths, myositis ossificans, elastofibroma dorsi, and extra-abdominal desmoid tumors are examples of primary chest wall tumors. Secondary chest wall cancers develop as a result of metastasis from other organs.

The actual causation of chest wall tumors is currently unknown in the literature; however, postulates suggest that genetics, food, and lifestyle decisions may all have a role in the formation of these tumors.

Extra-abdominal desmoid tumors are a type of aggressive fibromatosis that can appear at the site of a previous thoracotomy.

Research has not established the frequency of chest wall tumors in males versus females. The age of presentation varies; however, younger patients have smaller and more benign tumors, whereas older patients tend to have larger and more aggressive tumors.

The primary chest wall tumors have an incidence of less than two percent of the population. Chest wall neoplasms are either primary or metastatic, with a malignancy rate of about fifty percent, and either symptomatic or asymptomatic, with about twenty percent found incidentally on chest radiographs. Primary chest wall tumors represent five percent of all thoracic neoplasms.

The sarcomas of the chest wall form in the cartilage, soft tissues, and bones of the chest cavity, including chondrosarcomas, osteosarcomas, rhabdomyosarcomas, plasmacytomas, malignant fibrous histiocytomas, and Ewing sarcomas. The most common primary malignant chest wall tumors are chondrosarcomas.

Approximately fifty to eighty percent of chest wall tumors are malignant, and fifty-five percent of these arise from bone or cartilage and forty-five percent from soft tissue. Overall five-year survival after resection of primary chest wall neoplasms is approximately sixty percent. Recurrence can occur in up to fifty percent of patients, with a resultant five-year survival of seventeen percent.

There are two forms of chest wall tumors:

1. **Benign Tumours**: There are a few sub-categories of Chest Wall Benign Tumors, which are thoroughly detailed below:

A) OSTEOCHONDROMA:-

The most prevalent type of benign bone tumor is osteochondroma, which is found in the femur, humerus, and tibia [1]. However, osteochondromas in the chest are most common in the rib or scapula, where they are frequently detected near the costochondral junction, and they develop from aberrant growth of normal tissue [2]. Osteochondromas account for half of all benign rib tumors [3]. As the growth of bone exostoses progresses, these masses frequently cause pain [1]. Chondromas are cartilaginous tumors that usually appear near the sternocostal junction [4]. They are rather frequent, accounting for 15 to 20% of benign chest wall lesions. Chondromas are normally painless, slow growing, and appear between the ages of 20 and 30 [4]. Because distinguishing between chondroma and low-grade chondrosarcoma is difficult, all chondromas are included. It is treated as malignant lesions and wide excision is recommended [4].

SIGNS & SYMPTOMS:-

The patient will largely complain of acute discomfort from bony lesions on the chest wall. In addition, the patient reports bone deformity, loss of motion, and neurovascular compression.

Pneumothorax, hemothorax, pericardial injury, diaphragmatic injury, and other complications can occur in patients with chest wall osteochondroma [5].

PATHOPHYSIOLOGY:-

HME, a pediatric, autosomal-dominant condition with reported occurrences of 1 in 50,000 people globally, is characterized by the production of multiple osteochondromas. Patients with HME have autosomal dominant functional mutations in the EXT1 and/or EXT2 genes, which cause numerous osteochondromas to develop. Frame shift, missense, and splice-site mutations are examples of EXT mutations [5] The human EXT1 and EXT2 genes encode type II transmembrane glycoproteins that are found in the endoplasmic reticulum and are involved in glycosyltransferase activity [6]. Exostosin 1 (EXT1) and exostosin 2 (EXT2) glycosyltransferases form a stable hetero-oligomeric complex that accumulates in the Golgi apparatus and is involved in heparan sulfate proteoglycan (HSPG) biosynthesis [12].

HSPGs consist of extracellular core proteins in which a tetrasaccharide linker is synthesized on conserved serine residues of the core protein of HSPGs. EXT1 and EXT2 allow the elongation of heparan sulfate (HS) chains by sequentially adding alternating units of N-acetylglucosamine and glucuronic acid. As HS chains are created, deacetylation, sulfation, and epimerization occur [7]. Four HSPG isoform families have been identified: syndecan, glypican, perlecan, and CD44 [6]. Glypicans and syndecans that carry long HS chains specifically bind and interact with signaling proteins, plasma proteins, and growth factors. Therefore, these HSPGs affect a variety of neighboring cell responses, such as cell differentiation, cell-to-cell interaction, receptor trafficking, and control tissue morphogenesis and gradients of growth factors, such as fibroblast growth factors, bone morphogenetic proteins (BMPs), hedgehogs (HHs), and Wnts in the extracellular matrix [7]. The pathogenesis of osteochondroma development has not been clearly elucidated; however, HS synthesis deficiency most likely underlies the molecular mechanism of osteochondroma formation [6].

DIAGNOSIS:-

There are multiple modalities by which this can be diagnosed. The following methods are:-

PRESENTATION:-

Osteochondroma of the rib is exceedingly rare [9,10,11]. They may present as a swelling in the chest wall or as an incidental finding on the chest radiograph. Osteochondroma usually presents in childhood or adolescence. About 3% of solitary osteochondromas have vertebral and costal origin while they have been said to occur in 7% of individuals with hereditary multiple exostoses. Only 10% of rib tumors are benign and osteochondromas, the most common benign bone tumor, account for half of these [12]. The tumor occurs more frequently in men, with a male/female ratio of 3:1. Osteochondromas begin in childhood and grow until completion of skeletal maturity.

IMAGING:-

Plain radiography is sufficient to diagnose the typical side of osteochondroma. However, in certain bones such as the scapula, plain radiography could be a limitation of diagnosis. A CT scan is useful to diagnose these bones [8].

TREATMENT:-

Due to the growth of the chest wall lesion and the significant discomfort that the patient experienced, surgical resection of the main chest lesion with chest wall reconstruction [13].

(B) **CHONDROMAS:-**

Chondromas are typically found at the sternocostal junction arising from cartilaginous tissue[2] They are relatively common, making up 15 to 20% of benign chest wall lesions. Chondromas are usually painless, slow growing, and present between 20 and 30 years of age. The distinction between chondroma and low-grade chondrosarcoma is difficult, therefore all chondromas are treated as malignant lesions, and wide excision is recommended [4].

SIGNS & SYMPTOMS:-

- Chest pain

- Swelling in the chest
- A mass or lump protruding from the chest
- Muscle atrophy
- Impaired movement [14]

PATHOPHYSIOLOGY:-

In bone, chondromas may be classified as <u>enchondromas</u> (arising in the medullary cavity) and ecchondromas (arising in other skeletal cartilages) [10]. Chondromas are smooth, circumscribed, sometimes encapsulated, expansile masses composed of multilobulated, blue-white or white, cartilaginous tissue. In some masses, there may be areas of gelatinous (myxoid) material [15].

IMAGING:-

Imaging methods like chest wall radiography, CT scan & MRI is used to diagnose the tumour. Along with that biopsy is also used [8].

TREATMENT:-

Due to the growth of the chest wall lesion and the significant discomfort that the patient experienced, surgical resection of the main chest lesion with chest wall reconstruction [13].

(C) **FIBROUS DYSPLASIA:-**

Fibrous dysplasia typically appears in the lateral or posterior tract of the ribs and is the third most frequent benign chest wall lesion [3]. Normal bone is replaced with fibrous tissue forming a slow-growing mass.

SIGNS & SYMPTOMS:-

Fibrous dysplasia usually produces no symptoms. The lesions are detected accidentally during radiological investigations. However, in rare cases, they may become symptomatic as they grow in size. They can also cause pathologic fractures, neuropathy, and deformities [16].

PATHOPHYSIOLOGY:-

Fibrous Dysplasia is a developmental abnormality caused by a GS alpha protein mutation that leads to failure of the production of normal lamellar bone.

The condition usually presents in patients who are less than 30 years of age with an asymptomatic lesion that is found incidentally on radiographs.

DIAGNOSIS:-

Diagnosis is made with radiographs showing a lesion with ground glass appearance or a "punched-out" lesion with a well-defined margin of sclerotic bone.

IMAGING:-

Clinical, radiological, and histopathological investigations are the pillars for the diagnosis of fibrous dysplasia. CT scan findings are the cornerstone of radiologic evaluations. The "ground-glass" appearance is the result of medullary space replacement by the mixture of woven bone and fibrous components [17]. Polymerase chain reaction (PCR) can be utilized for the diagnosis. Missense point mutations in the Gsα at the Arg201 codon are positive and the tumor cells do not express the proliferating cell nuclear antigen [18]. Histologic features consist of cellular fibrous dysplasia containing a proliferation of bland and uniform spindle cells with sparse mitotic activity [19].

TREATMENT:-

Treatment is usually nonoperative with bisphosphonates for pain control. Surgical management is indicated for lesions that lead to bone deformities such as scoliosis or coxa vara.

Surgical intervention is indicated when symptomatic lesions or deformities and pathologic fractures are present. Regarding skeletal maturity and the possibility of tumor progression and maturation, age is an important factor in decision-making for surgical treatment [20, 21].

Complete resection of the lesion is sufficient and the defect has to be reconstructed.

(D) LIPOMAS:-

Lipoma is a mesenchymal tumor originating from fat cells [22]. It can be superficial or deep. Superficial lipoma is a common subcutaneous mass, usually benign and encapsulated, and composed almost entirely of fat [23]. Instead, deep lipoma and, especially, intramuscular lipoma (IL), a deep-seated lipoma that originates within the muscle, is extremely rare [24,25]. It should be assessed carefully, as it is more likely to be malignant and should be considered a well-differentiated liposarcoma until proven otherwise [26]. Indeed, Fletcher et al found that 83% presented infiltrative histopathologic features [27].

SIGNS & SYMPTOMS:-

Usually, it is a slowly growing asymptomatic mass. Pain is a late and uncommon symptom, usually in deep and very large IL due to the expansion of adjacent soft tissues or compression of the adjacent peripheral nerve [28].

PATHOPHYSIOLOGY:-

Patients often complain of a soft, mobile mass of tissue they can feel under the skin. These are typically painless unless they encroach joints, nerves, or blood vessels.

A genetic link has been demonstrated that cites that about two-thirds of lipomas exhibit genetic abnormalities. In a subgroup of lipomas, the *HMGA2* gene (located on 12q14.3) was involved in tumor pathogenesis.

Lipomas are composed of adipose/fat tissue, are mobile, soft to the touch, typically painless, and present subcutaneously. These are surrounded by a thin, fibrous capsule that is not attached to the underlying muscle fascia. In their typical form, they rarely present a diagnostic challenge [7]. These masses are typically less than 2 inches wide but may be larger.

On gross examination, the majority of ILs are seemingly circumscribed, masses of uniform, yellowish adipose tissue with mottled tan areas, and a soft consistency. Histologically, ILs have a relatively uniform appearance characterized by mature uni vacuolated adipocytes of fairly uniform size and shape, which irregularly infiltrate between muscle fibers and, in many places, completely replace the muscle bundles. They do not display nuclear atypia and there is no increased mitosis, hyperchromasia, pleomorphism, or multinucleation of fat cells [16].

IMAGING:-

CT and MRI are the most useful diagnostic methods to identify and mark out this mass and to reveal IL characteristics, such as size, locations, and relationship with neighboring structures to choose the best treatment. CT scan appearance of ILs reveals a hypodense mass situated within the muscle with Hounsfield values in the negative range. Attenuation is similar to that of fat tissue. The shape of the mass may vary but is usually ovoid or fusiform. The mass may be well circumscribed or have poorly defined margins. Thick and thin soft tissue density streaks are commonly found inside the lesion. The thickness of the streaks varies and they are interrupted occasionally. MRI is very useful in distinguishing fat-containing tumors from other soft tissue tumors. MRI is also an excellent imaging modality to distinguish among lipomatous masses. The fatty tissue in the ILs demonstrates high signal intensity on both T1- and T2-weighted images. Fat-suppressed sequences demonstrate signal suppression similar to normal fat. ILs can be homogeneous with intensity similar to subcutaneous fat or heterogeneous with intermingled muscle fibers and other types of tumor tissue [29, 30]. Ultrasonography instead is important to define the fatty nature of the lesion although it does not offer sufficient knowledge about the relationship with adjacent structures [22, 31, 32].

TREATMENT:-

Surgical excision is the best method to treat chest wall lipoma but encapsulation must be effectively removed so that recurrence is reduced [8]. If the decision is made to excise lipomas, then it should be done while the lesions are smaller rather than after they grow larger to reduce the risk of this encroaching on joints, nerves, and blood vessels, thus making the excision more difficult and invasive [8].

References:-

1. Tomo H, Ito Y, Aono M, Takaoka K. Chest wall deformity associated with osteochondroma of the scapula: a case report and review of the literature. *J Shoulder Elbow Surg.* 2005;14:103–106. [PubMed] [Google Scholar]

2. Tateishi U, Gladish G W, Kusumoto M, et al. Chest wall tumors: radiologic findings and pathologic correlation: part 1. Benign tumors. *Radiographics.* 2003;23:1477–1490. [PubMed] [Google Scholar]

3. Incarbone M, Pastorino U. Surgical treatment of chest wall tumors. *World J Surg.* 2001;25:218–230. [PubMed] [Google Scholar]

4. Shah A A, D'Amico T A. Primary chest wall tumors. *J Am Coll Surg.* 2010;210:360–366. [PubMed] [Google Scholar]

5. Shackcloth M J, Page R D. Scapular osteochondroma with reactive bursitis presenting as a chest wall tumour. *Eur J Cardiothorac Surg.* 2000;18:495–496. [PubMed] [Google Scholar]

6. Eroglu A, Kürkçüoglu I C, Karaoglanoglu N. Solitary eosinophilic granuloma of sternum. *Ann Thorac Surg.* 2004;77:329–331. [PubMed] [Google Scholar]

7. Bayram A S, Köprücüoglu M, Filiz G, Gebitekin C. Case of solitary eosinophilic granuloma of the sternum. *Thorac Cardiovasc Surg.* 2008;56:117–118. [PubMed] [Google Scholar]
8. Tungdim PH, Singh II, Mukherjee S, et al. Excision of solitary osteochondroma on the ventral aspect of left scapula presenting as pseudowinging in a 4-year-old boy: a rare case report. *J Orthop Case Rep* 2017;7:36–40. [PMC free article] [PubMed] [Google Scholar]
9. Kikuchi R, Mino N, Matsukura T, Hirai T. Resected osteochondroma of the rib in an elderly patient. *Gen Thorac Cardiovasc Surg.* 2010;58:588–91. [PubMed] [Google Scholar]
10. Tateishi U, Gladish GW, Kusumoto M, Hasegawa T, Yokoyama R, Tsuchiya R, et al. Chest wall tumors: radiologic findings and pathologic correlation: part 1. benign tumors. *Radiogra- phics.* 2003;23:1477–90. [PubMed] [Google Scholar]
11. Lee CY, Ham SY, Oh YW, Lee SH, Kim KT. Osteochondroma arising from a rib mimicking a calcifying anterior mediastinal mass. *J Korean Radiol Soc.* 2007;57:533–5. [Google Scholar]
12. Pairolero PC. Chest Wall Tumors. In: Shields TW, editor. *General Thoracic Surgery.* 4th ed. Vol. 579. Malvern, PA: Williams & Wilkins; 1994. [Google Scholar]
13. Alshehri A. Chest wall osteochondroma resection with biologic acellular bovine dermal mesh reconstruction in pediatric hereditary multiple exostoses: A case report and review of literature. *World J Clin Cases* 2023; 11(17): 4123-4132 [PMID: 37388792 DOI: 10.12998/wjcc.v11.i17.4123]
14. https://www.brighamandwomens.org/lung-center/diseases-and-conditions/chest-wall-cancer
15. Derek C. Knottenbelt OBE BVM&S DVM&S Dip ECEIM MRCVS, Janet C. Patterson-Kane BVSc PhD Dip ACVP MRCVS, Katie L. Snalune BSc MA VetMB Cert EM (Int.Med.) Cert ES (Soft Tissue) MRCVS

16. Favus M.D. *Harrison's principles of internal medicine.* 2005. Paget disease and other dysplasias of bone; pp. 2284–2285. [Google Scholar]

17. Singer F.R. Fibrous dysplasia of bone: the bone lesion unmasked. *Am. J. Pathol. [Internet]* 1997 Dec;**151**(6):1511–1515. http://www.ncbi.nlm.nih.gov/pubmed/9403700 Available from. [PMC free article] [PubMed] [Google Scholar]

18. 17. Maki M., Saitoh K., Horiuchi H., Morohoshi T., Fukayama M., Machinami R. Comparative study of fibrous dysplasia and osteofibrous dysplasia: histopathological, immunohistochemical, argyrophilic nucleolar organizer region and DNA ploidy analysis. *Pathol. Int.* 2001 Aug;**51**(8):603–611. http://www.ncbi.nlm.nih.gov/pubmed/11564214 Available from. [PubMed] [Google Scholar]

19. Aydın O., Barış S., Kefeli M., Şenel A., Yıldız L., Kandemir B. Fibröz Displazi(Olgu Bildirimi) *Journal of Experimental and Clinical Medicine.* 2009;**22**:156–159. Ondokuz Mayıs Üniversitesi. [Google Scholar]

20. Fitzpatrick K.A., Taljanovic M.S., Speer D.P., Graham A.R., Jacobson J.A., Barnes G.R., et al. Imaging findings of fibrous dysplasia with histopathologic and intraoperative correlation. *AJR Am. J. Roentgenol. [Internet]* 2004 Jun;**182**(6):1389–1398. http://www.ncbi.nlm.nih.gov/pubmed/15149980 Available from. [PubMed] [Google Scholar]

21. 12. Zhibin Y., Quanyong L., Libo C., Jun Z., Hankui L., Jifang Z., et al. The role of radionuclide bone scintigraphy in fibrous dysplasia of bone. *Clin. Nucl. Med. [Internet]* 2004 Mar;**29**(3):177–180. http://www.ncbi.nlm.nih.gov/pubmed/15162988 Available from. [PubMed] [Google Scholar]

22. S. Mc Tighe, I. Chernev,Orthop Rev, 6 (4) (2014), p. 5618Intramuscular lipoma: a review of the literature

23. C. Fletcher, Diagnostic Histopathology of Tumors (4th ed.), Elsevier (2014),Tumors of soft tissue

24. M. Murphey, J.F. Carroll, D.J. Flemming, T.L. Pope, F.H. Gannon, M.J. Kransdorf, Radiographics, 24 (5) (2004), pp. 1433-1466, From the archives of the AFIP: benign musculoskeletal lipomatous lesions

25. R.D. Di Subba, A. Suhny, H.C. Jonathan,(1st edition), Elsevier (2019) Problem solving in chest imaging

26. J. Nishida, T. Morita, A. Ogose, K. Okada, H. Kakizaki, T. Tajino, et al.,*J Orthop Sci, 12 (6) (2007), pp. 533-541,*Imaging characteristics of deep-seated lipomatous tumors: intramuscular lipoma, intermuscular lipoma, and lipoma-like liposarcoma

27. C.D. Fletcher, E. Martin-Bates,Histopathology, 12 (3) (1998), pp. 275-287Intramuscular and intermuscular lipoma: neglected diagnoses.

28. L. Ferrari, P. Haynes, J. Mack, G.S. Di Felice,Orthopedics, 32 (8) (2009)Intramuscular lipoma of the supraspinatus causing impingement syndrome

29. J. Nishida, H. Kakizaki, T. Tajino, M. Hatori, H. Orui, S. Ehara, et al.,*J Orthop Sci, 12 (6) (2007), pp. 533-541*Imaging characteristics of deep-seated lipomatous tumors: intramuscular lipoma, intermuscular lipoma, and lipoma-like liposarcoma

30. K. Matsumoto, S. Hukuda, M. Ishizawa, T. Chano, H. Okabe,Skeletal Radiol, 28 (3) (1999), pp. 145-152MRI findings in intramuscular lipomas

31. H. Berquist, R. Ehman, B. King, C. Hodgman, D. Ilstrup,Am J Roentgenol, 155 (6) (1990), pp. 1251-1255,Value of MR imaging in differentiating benign from malignant soft-tissue masses: study of 95 lesions

32. P. Inampudi, J.A. Jacobson, D.P. Fessell, R.C. Carlos, S.V. Patel, L.O. Delaney-Sathy, et al.,*Radiology, 233 (3) (2004), pp. 763-*

*767*Soft-tissue lipomas: accuracy of sonography in diagnosis with pathologic correlation

33. Silistreli OK, Durmuş EU, Ulusal BG, Oztan Y, Görgü M. What should be the treatment modality in giant cutaneous lipomas? Review of the literature and report of 4 cases. Br J Plast Surg. 2005 Apr;58(3):394-8. [PubMed]

34. HATCH DANIEL MD Fibrous Dysplasia,2021 June 21.

MALIGNANT TUMOURS:-

There are a few sub-categories of Chest Wall Malignant Tumors, which are thoroughly detailed below:

(A) SARCOMAS:-

When a tumor forms in the bones, soft tissue, or cartilage, and is malignant, we call it a sarcoma. Malignant chest wall tumors include many types of sarcoma. Symptoms of chest wall sarcomas vary with the tumor's classification and severity. The patient might experience difficulty breathing as well as pain and swelling surrounding the tumor.

The different forms of chest wall sarcomas are:-

1. CHONDROSARCOMA:-

Forms in cartilage and is the most common type of primary chest wall bone cancer.

SIGNS & SYMPTOMS:-

The patient may notice a painfully growing lump. Pain is the most common presenting symptom, with 95% of patients reporting it. The pain is frequently subtle and progressive, lasting 1 to 2 years prior to presentation. The discomfort is often reported as aching during the day and becoming worse, sometimes severe, at night. At the time of presentation, 30% to 80% of patients have a palpable soft tissue mass or fullness. In 3% to 17% of patients, pathologic fractures are the presenting symptom [3].

PATHOPHYSIOLOGY:-

Chondrosarcomas are malignant tumors that produce a chondroid matrix. Primary chondrosarcomas arise de novo. Secondary chondrosarcomas occur in preexisting benign cartilaginous neoplasms, such as a complication of a preexisting enchondroma or osteochondroma [1, 2]. Tumors that arise in the medullary cavity are considered central, or conventional intramedullary, chondrosarcomas, while those that occur near the surface of bone are referred to as peripheral, or juxtacortical. Primary chondrosarcoma is the third most common primary malignant tumor of bone, but the most common primary neoplasm involving the chest wall [3]. Ten percent of chondrosarcomas are radiation-induced [3]. A wide variety of primary neoplasms are associated with radiation-induced chondrosarcoma, as follows: Hodgkin's lymphoma, breast adenocarcinoma, squamous cell carcinoma of the larynx, thyroid carcinoma, non–small cell lung carcinoma, and retinoblastoma [4–10]. This particular case was felt to represent a primary chondrosarcoma.

Chondrosarcomas tend to be bulky tumors. Most are >4 cm in diameter, and some grow as large as 25 or 35 cm.

Permeation of bone, size, and periosteal invasion are specific findings of chondrosarcoma. Cellularity, nuclear atypia (including multinucleated cells), and increased proliferation (>10%) are all indicators of increasing grade and aggressive behavior. Apart from the typical chondrosarcomas, there are some rare types of this tumor including dedifferentiated chondrosarcoma, mesenchymal chondrosarcoma, clear cell chondrosarcoma, and myxoid chondrosarcoma. These rare forms are more aggressive and malignant [15]. Chondrosarcomas associated with clinical syndromes were previously discussed.

IMAGING:-

a) CHEST WALL RADIOGRAPHY:-. The classic radiographic appearance of chondrosarcoma is a lobulated, mixed lytic, and sclerotic lesion. The sclerotic regions on radiographs correspond to chondroid matrix mineralization. In more advanced stages, the mass becomes lobulated with endosteal scalloping and eventual cortical disruption and extension to the adjacent soft tissues. Higher-grade chondrosarcomas contain a relatively less extensive chondroid matrix. Well-organized calcific rings within cartilage usually signify a low-grade tumor. High-grade chondrosarcomas may contain more myxoid material and are frequently associated with large areas of noncalcified tumor matrix. When calcification occurs in high-grade chondrosarcomas, it tends to be amorphous, scattered, punctuate, or irregular [11]. The degree of endosteal scalloping is considered the best predictor in distinguishing chondrosarcoma from benign enchondroma on radiographs.

b) CT SCAN:-CT is optimal for the detection and characterization of the chondroid matrix, which classically has well-formed rings and arcs of mineralization. It also represents internal water content. Deep endosteal scalloping and soft tissue expansion, which are both considered aggressive features are also observed.

c) MRI:-MRI is the ideal modality to evaluate the extent of bone marrow involvement and extraosseous extension.

d) PET:- PET is highly sensitive in detecting high-grade chondrosarcoma metastasis. PET can be useful in optimizing the biopsy approach and targeting regions of the highest measured metabolic activity.

TREATMENT:-

The natural history and prognosis of chondrosarcoma is extremely variable. Overall 5-year survival rates for grade 1 chondrosarcomas are 90% to 94%, while those for grade 3 are 43% to 44%. For grade 1 chondrosarcomas with intact cortex and absence of soft tissue mass, consideration can be given to an intralesional procedure such as curettage with adjunctive ablation. However, if there are aggressive imaging features such as cortical breakthrough or soft tissue mass, or if the tumor is grade 2 or higher, wide surgical excision is required [3].

A Scandinavian study evaluated 106 consecutive chondrosarcomas involving the rib and sternum. The pathologic specimens were reviewed and graded 1 to 4, and the surgical margins were defined as wide, marginal, or intralesional. After wide surgical excision, the 10-year survival rate was 92%, and the local recurrence rate was 4%. In contrast, the 10-year survival rate was 47% and the local recurrence rate was 73% in patients treated with an intralesional approach. Prognostic factors for local recurrence included both surgical margins and histologic grade [17].

Due to the slow growth rate of chondrosarcomas—as supported by a low proliferation index with the Mib-1/Ki-67 proliferation marker—chondrosarcomas are known to be relatively radioresistant. Doses exceeding 60 Gy are recommended for effective treatment, which is often not tolerable for adjacent structures (e.g., neurologic tissue)[1, 12].

Other treatment approaches have included particle therapy with protons, which offers the advantage of a minimal exit dose after energy deposits within the tissue, thus effectively sparing adjacent structures [2]. Additionally, proton radiotherapy has proven beneficial in the setting of incompletely resected chondrosarcomas present at the skull base and axial skeleton, with reported local control rates of 85% to 100% [14]. Another documented approach is the use of radiotherapy with carbon ions, providing the physical advantages of proton therapy combined with higher radiobiologic activity. Local control rates with this approach are 96% and 90% at 3 and 4 years, respectively [2].

Chondrosarcomas present several architectural and structural barriers to systemic chemotherapy. In addition to their low proliferation index, they have poor vascularity and an abundant extracellular matrix that makes tumor perfusion difficult. Further, it is hypothesized that the expression of the multidrug-resistance 1 gene (P-glycoprotein), which confers resistance to doxorubicin, offers another explanation for the relative ineffectiveness of chemotherapeutic regimens [2]. There is no suggestion of benefit for low-grade chondrosarcomas with adjuvant chemotherapy, even in the metastatic setting. However, chemotherapy may have some role to play in the treatment of tumors of dedifferentiated and mesenchymal subtypes (especially with increased small blue cells). This latter type of chondrosarcoma is especially chemotherapy-sensitive, and tumor responses to conventional treatments have been noted. Specifically, Huvos et al [15] reported a median survival of 37.9 months, with a 50% 3-year survival, 42% 5-year survival, and 28% 10-year survival in a study of 32 patients. Cisplatin and Adriamycin–based regimens seem to have the most efficacy. Investigational classes of drugs including tyrosine kinase inhibitors, hormonal therapies, and angiogenesis inhibitors are also being studied [12]. Thus, no standardized proven approach exists for adjuvant chemotherapy in the setting of chondrosarcoma.

2. **RHABDOMYOSARCOMA**:

Rhabdomyosarcoma, the most common soft tissue sarcoma of children, has traditionally been classified into embryonal rhabdomyosarcoma (ERMS) and alveolar rhabdomyosarcoma (ARMS) for pediatric oncology practice. This review outlines the historical development of the classification of childhood rhabdomyosarcoma and the challenges that have been associated with it, particularly problems with the diagnosis of "solid variant" ARMS and its distinction from ERMS. In addition to differences in clinical presentation and outcome, a number of genetic features underpin the separation of ERMS from ARMS [18].

SIGNS & SYMPTOMS:-

Rhabdomyosarcoma is generally an asymptomatic mass or has symptoms associated with primary lesions. Patients present with pain due to the compression effect of neural structures by the mass[19, 20].

PATHOPHYSIOLOGY:-

PRMS is a common subtype in adults, where large pleomorphic rhabdomyoblasts are found with eosinophilic cytoplasm. Three morphological variants were found: classical, round cell, and spindle cell. Mixed types include a combination of more than one histological subtype. Establishing a diagnosis based on histopathology examination is difficult, so an experienced pathologist is essential [21]. The European Cooperative Group (COG), previously known as the Intergroup Rhabdomyosarcoma Study Group (IRSG), categorizes patients into four risk groups depending on the clinical staging system: Low risk, standard risk, high-risk, and very high risk. With 83% survival rates on stage I, 70% on stage II, 52% on stage III, and 20% on stage IV. The absence of distant metastases, favorable anatomic locations, total tumor removal when surgery and tumor size less than 5 cm are useful prognostic factors. As explained above, the outcome for rhabdomyosarcoma cases is worse in adults than in children due to a small number of cases and protocols that are not standardized. With a 5-year overall survival rate is 27% in adults [21].

DIAGNOSIS:-

All RMS patients require a complete laboratory examination, including total blood count, electrolytes, liver function tests, and renal function tests. Imaging of the primary lesion should be done with CT-scan or MRI. Imaging will determine the location of the tumor against vital structures and determine the size of the tumor. This parameter is an essential feature in determining operating actions. On physical examination, found a lump in the left chest wall. CT scan shows a soft tissue tumor in the anteromedial of the chest wall attached to the left lung [22].

Specific immunohistochemical markers for skeletal muscle differentiation help in the diagnosis of pleomorphic RMS. PRMS is found in at least one specific skeletal muscle marker (myoglobin, MyoD1 nucleus, myf4 nucleus, fast myosin) and nonspecific markers (desmin, myogenin). Myoglobin (95%) and skeletal muscle myosin (80%) are sensitive markers for PMRS.

TREATMENT:-

Chest wall rhabdomyosarcoma is normally treated with a combination of surgery, chemotherapy, and, in rare cases, radiation therapy. The stage of the disease and individual patient characteristics define the specific treatment approach. Early detection and therapy are critical for improving outcomes in patients with rhabdomyosarcoma of the chest wall [18].

3. **EWING'S SARCOMA**:-

Ewing's sarcoma in the chest wall is commonly referred to as "chest wall Ewing's sarcoma" because it begins in the bones or soft tissues of the chest wall. This type of Ewing's sarcoma shares many characteristics with other types of Ewing's sarcoma, but its position within the chest wall can provide distinct challenges and considerations [23].

SIGNS & SYMPTOMS:-

the chest wall Localized pain, swelling, soreness, and a palpable lump or mass in the chest wall are all symptoms of Ewing's sarcoma. Patients may also have symptoms associated with adjacent structural compression, which can result in breathing difficulties or other chest-related symptoms [24].

PATHOPHYSIOLOGY:-

The pathological segment demonstrates small fragments of tumor tissue composed of a proliferation of small, round, blue cells arranged in a solid pattern with the formation of occasional, vague rosettes. Areas of tumor necrosis can present. Scant cytoplasm and fine chromatin may be noted with infrequent mitotic figures. The immunohistochemistry is positive for CD99 (membranous) and NKX2.2 (nuclear) and was negative for PHOX2B, desmin, CD20,

CD45, synaptophysin, chromogranin, GFAP, SALL4, and myogenin. FISH studies detected rearrangement of EWSR1 (22q12) in 60% of the cells, and fusion of EWSR1 and FLI1 (11q24) was detected [25, 26].

IMAGING:-

- X RAY:- A cough that persists for more than three weeks and less than eight is considered a subacute cough [27]. Subacute and chronic cough warrant further investigation, and obtaining a chest X-ray is an essential and cost-effective investigation modality.
- CT SCAN:- Ewing's sarcoma usually presents a single well-defined mass with an inhomogeneous appearance on chest CT scans. Calcifications and pleural effusions involving the affected side of the chest are seen. Additionally, these masses can extend to the chest wall and mediastinum with invasion and displacement of surrounding structures [28,29].
- BIOPSY:-Extensive necrosis seen in tissue biopsy is also a feature of Ewing's sarcoma, and the identification of t(11:22) translocation resulting in the EWS-FLI1 fusion gene is the characteristic feature [30]. EWSR1/FLI1 fusion is seen in approximately 95% of Ewing's sarcoma and is about 90% specific [25,26]

TREATMENT:-

Ewing's sarcoma of the thorax, also called Askin's tumor, is a rare entity classified within PNET by the World Health Organization [24]. Clinically, this often mimics pneumonia with fever, cough, chest pain, and shortness of breath [31]. Due to the rarity of the disease, there are no clear treatment protocols, but a combination of surgical removal of the tumor followed by radiation and combination chemotherapy with two to six drugs, including doxorubicin, actinomycin D, cyclophosphamide, ifosfamide, vincristine, etoposide, busulfan, melphalan, and carboplatin, has shown to improve the prognosis [32].

B) **PLASMACYTOMA:-**

Plasmacytomas of bone are defined as clonal proliferations of plasma cells identical to those of plasma cell myeloma, which manifest a localized osseous growth. Plasmacytomas can be divided into multiple, solitary osseous, and solitary extraosseous or extramedullary plasmacytomas and are rare as compared with multiple myeloma [33]. Localized SPB is a rare disease and is characterized by one or two isolated bone lesions with no evidence of disease dissemination [33].

SIGNS & SYMPTOMS:-

The symptoms of a chest wall plasmacytoma can vary but may include localized pain, swelling, tenderness, or a palpable mass in the chest wall. Depending on its size and location, the tumor can also cause pressure on nearby structures, leading to symptoms such as difficulty breathing or coughing.

PATHOPHYSIOLOGY:-

Plasmacytoma, first described by Schridde in 1905, is a rare entity and is defined as a localized mass of neoplastic monoclonal plasma cells [34]. They are not associated with systemic manifestations of MM and SPB is commoner than SEP.

DIAGNOSIS:-

The use of CT, MRI, or PET/CT in the evaluation of plasma cell dyscrasia has increased the chances of detecting multiple soft tissue or additional bone lesions, thus accurately diagnosing cases of MSP when biochemical and laboratory investigations are within normal limits [35, 36, 37].

SERUM PROTEIN's (SP) are usually diagnosed by lesional biopsy or fine needle aspiration technique. Flouroscopy-guided or CT-guided lesional biopsy of the spine can be performed. Keeping in mind the rarity of SPs, histopathological evaluation is mandatory for diagnosis as well as to rule out other differentials such as bone tumors and lymphomas [38]

TREATMENT:-

SPs are treated with either radiotherapy, surgery, or a combination of both. The option of treatment is site-specific with most SPB and SEP of the lower respiratory tract being managed with radiotherapy alone. SEPs of the upper respiratory system may require both radiotherapy and surgery, whereas, SEPs of the gastrointestinal tract require surgical excision [39].

(C) **MALIGNANT FIBROUS HISTIOCYTOMA:-**

Malignant fibrous histiocytoma (MFR) is a deep-seated pleomorphic sarcoma of adults, which occurs most frequently in the deep fascia and skeletal muscle of the extremities and trunk. A rare tumor, initially described in 1964 by O'Brien and Stout [40], who considered it to have a histiocytic origin, it has since been increasingly recognized as a discrete entity. Previously it had been confused with other poorly differentiated pleomorphic sarcomas.

SIGNS & SYMPTOMS:-

The symptoms of chest wall malignant fibrous histiocytoma may include pain, swelling, a palpable mass, and sometimes difficulty breathing or chest wall deformities. However, these symptoms can be non-specific and may resemble other chest wall conditions [41].

PATHOPHYSIOLOGY:-

MFH is a soft tissue sarcoma occurring principally in middle-aged individuals and situated in the deep tissues of the extremities and trunk. The tumor is characterized by a mixture of fibroblastic and histiocytic elements arranged in a storiform pattern and accompanied by giant cells and inflammatory cells. Because of the highly variable morphologic appearance, even within an individual tumor, diagnosis is difficult with small biopsy specimens [42, 43].

DIAGNOSIS:-

CT and magnetic resonance (MR) imaging are useful for the radiological evaluation of the soft tissue component. CT can provide more accurate detection of cortical bone destruction, whereas MRI displays the infiltration of the bone marrow and the extent of the mass with good resolution [44]. The mass usually shows intense enhancement on CT with a clear margin separating it from the surrounding tissue [45]. Furthermore, the mass often shows decreased central attenuation due to necrosis, hemorrhage, and mucoid material [46].

TREATMENT:-

Wide resection is the first choice treatment and additional chemotherapy may play a role in treating osseous MFH. A good response to preoperative chemotherapy seems to be associated with an excellent prognosis [47, 48]. Postoperative radiation therapy is essential in cases of tumors with positive surgical margins following wide complete gross excision [49].

References:-

1. Mazanet R, Antman KH. Sarcomas of soft tissue and bone. *Cancer.* 1991;68(3):463–473. [PubMed] [Google Scholar]

2. Cakir O, Topal U, Bayram AS, Tolunay S. Sarcomas: rare primary malignant tumors of the thorax. *Diagn Interv Radiol.* 2005;11(1):23–27. [PubMed] [Google Scholar]

3. Murphey MD, Walker EA, Wilson AJ, Kransdorf MJ, Temple HT, Gannon FH. From the archives of the AFIP: imaging of primary chondrosarcoma: radiologic-pathologic correlation. *Radiographics.* 2003;23(5):1245–1278. [PubMed] [Google Scholar]

4. Weatherby RP, Dahlin DC, Ivins JC. Postradiation sarcoma of bone: review of 78 Mayo Clinic cases. *Mayo Clin Proc.* 1981;56(5):294–306. [PubMed] [Google Scholar]

5. Sauter ER, Keller SM, Curran WJ, Russo J, Langer CJ. Radiation-induced chest-wall chondrosarcoma following surgical resection and radiotherapy for non-small-cell lung cancer. *J Natl Cancer Inst.* 1993;85(2):162–163. [PubMed] [Google Scholar]

6. Schwarz RE, Burt M. Radiation-associated malignant tumors of the chest wall. *Ann Surg Oncol.* 1996;3(4):387–392. [PubMed] [Google Scholar]

7. Mohammadianpanah M, Gramizadeh B, Omidvari SH, Mosalaei A. Radiation-induced chondrosarcoma of the maxilla 7-year after combined chemoradiation for tonsillar lymphoma. *J Postgrad Med.* 2004;50(3):200–201. [PubMed] [Google Scholar]

8. Fitzwater JE, Cabaud HE, Farr GH. Irradiation-induced chondrosarcoma. A case report. *J Bone Joint Surg Am.* 1976;58(7):1037–1039. [PubMed] [Google Scholar]

9. Peimer CA, Yuan HA, Sagerman RH. Postradiation chondrosarcoma. A case report. *J Bone Joint Surg Am.* 1976;58(7):1033–1036. [PubMed] [Google Scholar]

10. Sheppard DG, Libshitz HI. Post-radiation sarcomas: a review of the clinical and imaging features in 63 cases. *Clin Radiol.* 2001;56(1):22–29. [PubMed] [Google Scholar]

11. Resnick D, Niwayama G, editors. *Diagnosis of Bone and Joint Disorders.* 2nd ed. Philadelphia: Saunders; 1988. pp. 3897–3919. [Google Scholar]

12. Gelderblom H, Hogendoorn PC, Dijkstra SD, van Rijswijk CS, Krol AD, Taminiau AH, Bovée JV. The clinical approach towards chondrosarcoma. *Oncologist.* 2008;13(3):320–329. [PubMed] [Google Scholar]

13. Widhe B, Bauer HC, Scandinavian Sarcoma Group Surgical treatment is decisive for outcome in chondrosarcoma of the chest wall: a population-based Scandinavian Sarcoma Group study of 106 patients. *J Thorac Cardiovasc Surg.* 2009;137(3):610–614. [PubMed] [Google Scholar]

14. Hug EB, Loredo LN, Slater JD, DeVries A, Grove RI, Schaefer RA, Rosenberg AE, Slater JM. Proton radiation therapy for chordomas and chondrosarcomas of the skull base. *J Neurosurg.* 1999;91(3):432–439. [PubMed] [Google Scholar]

15. Huvos AG, Rosen G, Dabska M, Marcove RC. Mesenchymal chondrosarcoma. A clinicopathologic analysis of 35 patients with emphasis on treatment. *Cancer.* 1983;51(7):1230–1237. [PubMed] [Google Scholar]

16. Parham, D. M., & Barr, F. G. (2013). "Classification of rhabdomyosarcoma and its molecular basis." Advances in Anatomic Pathology, 20(6), 387-397.

17. Breneman, J. C., Wiener, E. S., Teot, L. A., et al. (2003). "Prognostic factors and clinical outcomes in children and adolescents with metastatic rhabdomyosarcoma—a report from the Intergroup Rhabdomyosarcoma Study IV." Journal of Clinical Oncology, 21(1), 78-84.

18. Little D.J., Ballo M.T., Zagars G.K., Pisters P.W., Patel S.R., El-Naggar A.K., Garden A.S., Benjamin R.S. Adult rhabdomyosarcoma: outcome following multimodality treatment. *Cancer.* 2002;**95**(2):377–388. doi: 10.1002/cncr.10669. [PubMed] [CrossRef] [Google Scholar]

19. Spalteholz Matthias, Gulow Jens. Pleomorphic rhabdomyosarcoma infiltrating thoracic spine in a 59-year-old female patient: Case report. *GMS Interdiscip. Plast. Reconstr. Surg. DGPW.* 2017;**6** [PMC free article] [PubMed] [Google Scholar]

20. Ruiz-Mesa Catalina. Rhabdomyosarcoma in adults: new perspectives on therapy. *Curr. Treat. Opt. Oncol.* 2015;**16** 2, s.l.: Springer. [Google Scholar]

21. Weiss S.W., Goldblum J.R. In: *Enzinger and Weiss's Soft Tissue Tumors. Rhabdomyosarcoma.* 5th ed. Weiss S.W., Goldblum J.R., editors. Elsevier; St. Louis: 2008. pp. 595–632. [Google Scholar]

22. Miettinen M. Rhabdomyosarcoma in patients older than 40 years of age. *Cancer.* 1988;**62**(9):2060–2065. [PubMed] [Google Scholar]

23. Changes in incidence and survival of Ewing sarcoma patients over the past 3 decades: Surveillance Epidemiology and End Results data. Esiashvili N, Goodman M, Marcus RB Jr. *J Pediatr Hematol Oncol.* 2008;30:425–430. [PubMed] [Google Scholar]

24. Askin tumor: case report and literature review. Cueto-Ramos RG, Ponce-Escobedo AN, Montero-Cantú CA, Muñoz-Maldonadoa GE, Ruiz-Holguínb E, Vilches-Cisnerosb N. *Medicina Universitaria.* 2015;17:213–217. [Google Scholar]

25. Ewing sarcoma fusion protein EWSR1/FLI1 interacts with EWSR1 leading to mitotic defects in zebrafish embryos and human cell lines. Embree LJ, Azuma M, Hickstein DD. *Cancer Res.* 2009;69:4363–4371. [PMC free article] [PubMed] [Google Scholar]

26. Molecular diagnosis in Ewing family tumors: the Rizzoli experience--222 consecutive cases in four years. Gamberi G, Cocchi S, Benini S, et al. *J Mol Diagn.* 2011;13:313–324. [PMC free article] [PubMed] [Google Scholar]

27. Diagnosis and management of cough executive summary: ACCP evidence-based clinical practice guidelines. Irwin RS, Baumann MH, Bolser DC, et al. *Chest.* 2006;129:1–23. [PMC free article] [PubMed] [Google Scholar]

28. Primary extraosseous Ewing sarcoma of the lung: case report and literature review. Shet N, Stanescu L, Deutsch G. *Radiol Case Rep.* 2013;8:832. [PMC free article] [PubMed] [Google Scholar]

29. Primary thoracic sarcomas. Gladish GW, Sabloff BM, Munden RF, Truong MT, Erasmus JJ, Chasen MH. *Radiographics.* 2002;22:621–637. [PubMed] [Google Scholar]

30. Ewing's sarcoma. Balamuth NJ, Womer RB. *Lancet Oncol.* 2010;11:184–192. [PubMed] [Google Scholar]

31. Askin's tumor: 11 cases and a review of the literature. Zhang KE, Lu R, Zhang P, Shen S, Li X. https://doi.org/10.3892/ol.2015.3902. *Oncol Lett.* 2016;11:253–256. [PMC free article] [PubMed] [Google Scholar]

32. Askin's tumor: a case report and literature review. Benbrahim Z, Arifi S, Daoudi K, et al. *World J Surg Oncol.* 2013;11:10. [PMC free article] [PubMed] [Google Scholar]

33. Ashiq Masood, Hudhud Kanan H, Hegazi AZ, Syed Gaffar. Mediastinal plasmacytoma with multiple myeloma presenting as a diagnostic dilemma. *Cases J.* 2008;1:116. [PMC free article] [PubMed] [Google Scholar]

34. Kose M, Buraniqi E, Akpinar TS, Kayacan S, Tukek T. Relapse of multiple myeloma presenting as extramedullary Plasmacytomas in multiple organs. *Case Rep Hematol.* 2015;**2015**:452305. doi: 10.1155/2015/452305. [PMC free article] [PubMed] [CrossRef] [Google Scholar]

35. Dattolo P., Allinovi M., Michelassi S., Pizzarelli F. Multiple solitary plasmacytoma with multifocal bone involvement. First clinical case report in a uraemic patient. *Case Reports.* 2013;**2013**(may23 1):bcr2013009157–bcr2013009157. [PMC free article] [PubMed] [Google Scholar]

36. Zhang L, Zhang X, He Q, Zhang R, Fan W. The role of initial 18F-FDG PET/CT in the management of patients with suspected extramedullary plasmacytoma. *Cancer Imaging.* 2018;**18**:19. doi: 10.1186/s40644-018-0152-x. [PMC free article] [PubMed] [CrossRef] [Google Scholar]

37. Ooi GC, Chim JC, Au WY, et al. Radiologic manifestations of primary solitary extramedullary and multiple solitary plasmacytomas. *AJR Am J Roentgenol.* 2006;**186**:821–827. doi: 10.2214/AJR.04.1787. [PubMed] [CrossRef] [Google Scholar]

38. Lim YH, Park SK, Oh HS, et al. A case of primary Plasmacytoma of lymph nodes. *Korean J Intern Med.* 2005;**20**:183–186. doi:

10.3904/kjim.2005.20.2.183. [PMC free article] [PubMed] [CrossRef] [Google Scholar]

39. Grammatico S, Scalzulli E, Petrucci MT. Solitary Plasmacytoma. *Mediterr J Hematol Infect Dis.* 2017;9(1):e2017052. doi: 10.4084/MJHID.2017.052. [PMC free article] [PubMed] [CrossRef] [Google Scholar]

40. O'Brien JE, Stout AP: Malignant fibrous xanthomas. Cancer 17:1445-1455, 1964

41. Mills SA, Breyer RH, Johnston FR, Hudspeth AS, Marshall RB, Choplin RH, Cordell AR, Myers RT: Malignant fibrous histiocytoma of the mediastinum and lung. A report of three cases. J THORAC CARDIOVASC SURG 84:367-372, 1982

42. Kern WH, Hughes RK, Meyer BW, Harley DP: Malignant fibrous histiocytoma of the lung. Cancer 44: 1793- 1801, 1979

43. Chowdhury LN, Swerdlow MA, Jao W, Kathpalia S, Desser RK: Post irradiation malignant fibrous histiocytoma of the lung, Demonstration of alpha I antitrypsin material in the neoplastic cells. Am J Clin Pathol 14:820- 826, 1980

44. Kuhlman JE, Bouchardy L, Fishman EK, Zerhouni EA. CT and MR imaging evaluation of chest wall disorders. *RadioGraphics.* 1994;14:571–595. [PubMed] [Google Scholar]

45. Tateishi U, Kusumoto M, Hasegawa T, Yokoyama R, Moriyama N. Primary malignant fibrous histiocytoma of the chest wall: CT and MR appearance. *J Comput Assist Tomogr.* 2002;26:558–563. [PubMed] [Google Scholar]

46. Munk PL, Sallomi DF, Janzen DL, Lee MJ, Connell DG, O'Connell JX, et al. Malignant fibrous histiocytoma of soft tissue imaging with emphasis on MRI. *J Comput Assist Tomogr.* 1998;22:819–826. [PubMed] [Google Scholar]

47. Dahlin DC, Unni KK. *Bone tumors: General Aspects and Data on 8,542 Cases.* 4th ed. Springfied: Thomas; 1986. [Google Scholar]

48. Bielack SS, Schroeders A, Fuchs N, Bacci G, Bauer HC, Mapeli S, et al. Malignant fibrous histiocytoma of bone: a retrospective EMSOS study of 125 cases. European Musculo-Skeletal Oncology Society. *Acta Orthop Scand.* 1999;70:353–360. [PubMed] [Google Scholar]

49. Belal A, Kandil A, Allam A, Khafaga Y, El-Husseiny G, El-Enbaby A, et al. Malignant fibrous histiocytoma: a retrospective study of 109 cases. *Am J Clin Oncol.* 2002;25:16–22. [PubMed] [Google Scholar]

Chapter 4
Clinical Presentations and Symptoms

Md Kaif Khan, Prof Parijat Suryavanshi

Introduction:

Identifying the clinical presentations and symptoms of chest wall tumors is pivotal for their diagnosis and management. These tumors can present in a multitude of ways, sometimes with subtle or nonspecific signs that may go unnoticed. It's crucial to be vigilant in recognizing the associated symptoms, as early detection is crucial for timely intervention. In this introduction, we will explore the diverse clinical presentations and symptoms that individuals might encounter when dealing with chest wall tumors, emphasizing the significance of thorough evaluation and accurate diagnosis to guide appropriate treatment approaches.

Detection of Chest Wall Masses:

Approximately one-fifth of chest wall masses are incidentally detected during unrelated medical imaging investigations [1].

Common Symptoms at Presentation:

The remaining four-fifths of cases present with a range of symptoms, including:

- Pain
- Dyspnea
- Neurologic involvement
- Vascular involvement [2].

Pain as a Symptom:

- Pain is a prominent symptom in chest wall tumor cases.

- Malignant tumors typically cause pain.

- Only two-thirds of benign tumors are associated with pain.

- However, pain alone is not a reliable indicator of malignancy [3].

Different Presentation Patterns:

- Chest wall tumors can present in various ways.

- Some patients remain asymptomatic until the tumor reaches an advanced stage.

- Notably, tumors of bone and cartilage origin tend to be painful [3].

- There are no definitive signs or symptoms that reliably distinguish between benign and malignant chest wall tumors [3].

Other Clinical Manifestations:

- Chest wall tumors can lead to additional clinical presentations, such as:

- Muscle weakness

- Atrophy in the upper extremities

- These symptoms may arise due to compression of the brachial plexus by the tumor [1].

Diagnostic Challenges:

- Heterogeneous Nature of Chest Wall Tumors:

- Chest wall tumors are an intriguing diagnostic puzzle due to their heterogeneous nature. They represent a diverse group of lesions that vary widely in pathology. These tumors can originate from any anatomical structure within the chest wall [5].
- Despite being relatively uncommon, chest wall tumors are known to challenge the diagnostic acumen of surgeons, making up less than 5% of thoracic malignancies [5].

Treatment Approach:

- The cornerstone of treatment for chest wall tumors is wide local excision. However, there is a critical distinction for malignant tumors, which often necessitate wider surgical margins to ensure complete removal. Adjuvant radiation therapy is typically recommended for cases with positive margins, highlighting the complexities of managing these tumors [5].
- When considering treatment options, it's crucial to recognize that chemotherapy rarely yields satisfactory results in the context of chest wall tumors [5].
- Local control emerges as a paramount prognostic factor. The presence of positive margins can severely limit disease-free survival. Therefore, surgeons aim for full oncologic resection, often striving for 4-cm margins to maximize therapeutic success [5].

Complexity of Resection and Reconstruction:

- The complexity of resection and reconstruction in chest wall tumor cases can vary widely. While small lesions generally permit straightforward surgical interventions, larger and more advanced tumors may pose considerable challenges [5].

Types of Primary Chest Wall Tumors:

- Primary chest wall tumors, though relatively rare, encompass a broad spectrum of neoplasms. They can arise not only from the bones or cartilage of the chest wall but also from surrounding subcutaneous tissues, muscles, and blood vessels [6]. These tumors can sometimes mimic benign conditions like lipomas or hematomas, complicating diagnosis [6].

- It's important to note that primary chest wall tumors encompass both benign and malignant neoplasms. They involve various chest wall components, such as muscle, fat, blood vessels, nerve sheaths, cartilage, and bone. Additionally, they may include metastatic tumors and local invasions originating from adjacent organs such as the lung, mediastinum, pleura, or breast [7].

Incidence and Sarcoma Prevalence:

- The incidence of primary chest wall tumors is relatively low, accounting for just 5% of all chest wall tumors [8].
- Notably, the majority of primary chest wall tumors fall into the category of sarcomas, constituting 15-20% of all sarcomas. These tumors are categorized according to the 4th edition of the World Health Organization (WHO) Classification [8].

Multidisciplinary Approach:

- Dealing with advanced chest wall tumors or cases requiring significant functional restoration often necessitates a multidisciplinary approach [5]. Collaboration among various specialists, including pathologists, thoracic surgeons, plastic surgeons, neurosurgeons, radiation medicine experts, oncologists, and physical medicine and rehabilitation specialists, is vital for comprehensive preoperative planning and successful patient management [5].

Staging:

Basis of Staging:

- Staging of chest wall tumors is primarily determined by two critical factors: the size of the tumor and its metastatic potential, i.e., whether it has the capacity to spread to nearby lymph nodes or other parts of the body [8].

Incidence and Predominance of Sarcomas:

- The incidence of primary chest wall tumors is relatively low, constituting just 5% of all chest wall tumors [8].

- It's worth noting that the majority of primary chest wall tumors fall into the category of sarcomas, comprising 15-20% of all sarcomas. These sarcomas are categorized according to the 4th edition of the World Health Organization (WHO) Classification [8].

Lack of TNM Staging for Chest Wall Sarcomas:

- Despite their significance, chest wall sarcomas present a unique challenge in terms of staging. Due to their low incidence and the limited availability of high-level clinical evidence, there is currently no established TNM (Tumor-Node-Metastasis) staging system specific to chest wall sarcomas [8].

- As a result, the staging of chest wall sarcomas relies on alternative criteria. Currently, the 8th edition TNM staging criteria for bone tumors (trunk, extremities, skull, and maxillofacial) and soft tissue sarcomas (trunk and extremities) are often referenced based on postoperative pathological diagnoses [9].

Prognostic Factors:

- Information regarding the treatment and prognosis of adult soft tissue sarcomas (STS) located in the chest wall is limited, particularly in cases involving full-thickness chest wall resection (CWR) [10].

- Existing series of patients are often collected over several decades, and it's important to note that some of these series may include children or adolescents with small-cell sarcomas, which typically require salvage surgery following chemotherapy [10].

Scarce Prognostic Data Beyond Tumor Grade:

- The current literature offers little in terms of prognostic factors beyond tumor grade. This underscores the need for additional research and analysis to provide surgeons with more comprehensive, evidence-based insights for their patients [11, 12].

- In our analysis, several negative prognostic factors were identified through univariate analysis, including pathological grade II/III, absence of sternal resection, and the absence of tumor invasion into bones confirmed by pathological examination. Tumor grade's role as a prognostic factor aligns with established knowledge in sarcoma surgery [11, 12].

- It's noteworthy that the reasons behind bone invasion and sternal resection as favorable prognostic factors remain unclear. It's possible that certain primary (non-osteo-) sarcomas of the bone exhibit better outcomes than soft tissue sarcomas [11, 12]. However, this retrospective study did not allow us to distinguish between primary bone sarcomas and other sarcomas [11, 12].

- Other factors that may influence prognosis include radical resection (particularly confirmed in our series for local recurrence-free survival in the clinical radical group), tumor size less than 5 cm, patient age (noted in our series for overall survival), synchronous metastases, and local recurrence. However, it's important to acknowledge that the prognostic significance of some of these factors may vary and require further validation [12-14].

Factors Considered in Prognostic Assessment:

- In the assessment of prognosis, various factors were considered, including: [15]
- Age at diagnosis
- Duration of symptoms
- Tumor size
- Tumor location

- Tumor depth
- Tumor grade
- Surgical margin
- Radiotherapy
- Calendar year of diagnosis
- Tumor size, recorded as the largest diameter (in cm) based on pathological specimens, was used as a determinant. In cases where surgical treatment was not administered or pathology reports were insufficient, diagnostic images were used to determine size.
- Tumors located in the shoulder and gluteal area were categorized as trunk tumors.
- Surgical margins were defined based on pathological specimens as intralesional/marginal if the incision was within the tumor or the pseudocapsule or as wide if the tumor was surrounded by a cuff of normal tissue.

References:

1- Shah AA, D'Amico TA. Primary chest wall tumors. Journal of the American College of Surgeons. 2010 Mar 1;210(3):360-6.

2- Yuh DD, Vricella LA, Yang SC, Doty JR. Johns Hopkins textbook of cardiothoracic surgery. (No Title). 2014 Feb 5

3- Athanassiadi K, Kalavrouziotis G, Rondogianni D, Loutsidis A, Hatzimichalis A, Bellenis I. Primary chest wall tumors: early and long-term results of surgical treatment. European Journal of cardio-thoracic surgery. 2001 May 1;19(5):589-93

5 - David EA, Marshall MB. Review of chest wall tumors: a diagnostic, therapeutic, and reconstructive challenge. InSeminars in plastic surgery 2011 Feb (Vol. 25, No. 01, pp. 016-024). © Thieme Medical Publishers

6- Gonfiotti A, Salvicchi A, Voltolini L. Chest-Wall Tumors and Surgical Techniques: State-of-the-Art and Our Institutional Experience. Journal of Clinical Medicine. 2022 Sep 20;11(19):5516

7- Smith SE, Keshavjee S. Primary chest wall tumors. Thoracic surgery clinics. 2010 Nov 1;20(4):495-507

8- Fletcher C, Bridge JA, Hogendoorn PC, Mertens F. WHO classification of tumours of soft tissue and bone: WHO classification of tumours, vol. 5. World Health Organization; 2013

9- Tanaka K, Ozaki T. New TNM classification (AJCC eighth edition) of bone and soft tissue sarcomas: JCOG Bone and Soft Tissue Tumor Study Group. Japanese journal of clinical oncology. 2019 Feb;49(2):103-7

10- van Geel AN, Wouters MW, Lans TE, Schmitz PI, Verhoef C. Chest wall resection for adult soft tissue sarcomas and chondrosarcomas: analysis of prognostic factors. World journal of surgery. 2011 Jan;35:63-9.

11- Pfannschmidt J, Geisbüsch P, Muley T, Dienemann H, Hoffmann H. Surgical treatment of primary soft tissue sarcomas involving the chest: experiences in 25 patients. The Thoracic and Cardiovascular Surgeon. 2006 Apr;54(03):182-7.

12- Gross JL, Younes RN, Haddad FJ, Deheinzelin D, Pinto CA, Costa ML. Soft-tissue sarcomas of the chest wall: prognostic factors. Chest. 2005 Mar 1;127(3):902-8.

13 Burt M, Fulton M, Wessner-Dunlap S, Karpeh M, Huvos AG, Bains MS, Martini N, McCormack PM, Rusch VW, Ginsberg RJ. Primary bony and cartilaginous sarcomas of chest wall: results of therapy. The Annals of thoracic surgery. 1992 Aug 1;54(2):226-32.

14 Perry RR, Venzon D, Roth JA, Pass HI. Survival after surgical resection for high-grade chest wall sarcomas. The Annals of thoracic surgery. 1990 Mar 1;49(3):363-9.

15 Maretty-Nielsen K, Aggerholm-Pedersen N, Safwat A, Jørgensen PH, Hansen BH, Baerentzen S, Pedersen AB, Keller J. Prognostic factors for local recurrence and mortality in adult soft tissue sarcoma of the extremities and trunk wall: a cohort study of 922 consecutive patients. Acta orthopaedica. 2014 Jun 1;85(3):323-32.

Chapter 5
Imaging Techniques, Tissue Biopsy, and Their Role in Chest Wall Tumor Diagnosis

Shubhajeet Roy, Md Kaif Khan, Dr Anurag Rai, Dr Shiv Rajan

Introduction:

Chest wall tumor diagnosis depends on a vital combination of advanced imaging techniques and tissue biopsy. These diagnostic tools are pivotal in precisely identifying and characterizing these chest wall tumors. In this introductory discussion, we'll explore the importance of imaging techniques and tissue biopsy in diagnosing chest wall tumors. Our exploration will put light on how these methods contribute to a holistic understanding of these conditions, ultimately enabling timely and effective patient management and various approaches.

Imaging Challenges and the Need for Tissue Biopsy

Chest wall tumors present a complex diagnostic challenge due to their significant histological diversity. Distinguishing between benign and malignant tumors remains elusive through radiological imaging alone [1]. Hence, tissue biopsy becomes indispensable to confirm the diagnosis [1].

Types of Tissue Biopsy

Pathological tissue samples are typically acquired through various biopsy techniques: fine-needle aspiration, incisional biopsy, or excisional biopsy [16]. Each method has its place in the diagnostic process.

1. Fine-Needle Aspiration: When metastatic lesions are suspected, fine-needle aspiration is often a reasonable choice. In fact, several studies suggest that core needle biopsy in bone tumors can provide diagnostic accuracy on par with incisional biopsy [16]. However, fine-needle aspiration's drawback is the limited tissue it yields, which can be insufficient for a definitive diagnosis [16].

2. Incisional Biopsy: For tumors exceeding 5 cm in size, an incisional biopsy is typically performed. However, it's essential to consider that when definitive surgical resection is planned, re-excision of the biopsy site becomes necessary [14].

3. Excisional Biopsy: On the other hand, for small lesions measuring less than 2 cm, an excisional biopsy might be the choice. In such cases, ensuring wide negative margins, typically at least 2 cm, is crucial. Importantly, an excisional biopsy serves a dual purpose, offering both diagnostic insights and therapeutic benefits [14].

Role of Imaging in Biopsy Planning

In the process of planning a biopsy, imaging techniques play a pivotal role. They guide the choice of biopsy method and provide critical insights into the tumor's characteristics and location.

1. Chest Radiography: This is frequently the initial step in the radiological evaluation of chest-wall tumors. Chest X-rays offer valuable information, such as the lesion's location, size, and specific characteristics like calcification, erosion, and bone destruction [14]. Some bone tumors of the chest wall even exhibit pathognomonic features that can be identified through chest X-rays. However, it's worth noting that early-stage tumors might not

be apparent on chest X-rays. Remarkably, in certain cases, conventional radiography alone can provide sufficient diagnostic information, obviating the need for invasive tissue biopsy [14].

2. <u>Computed Tomography (CT)</u>: CT imaging is instrumental in assessing chest-wall tumors due to its superior sensitivity and specificity compared to chest X-rays. CT also offers the advantage of enhanced image resolution, particularly when a contrast medium is used. This technique allows for a comprehensive evaluation, including an assessment of the tumor's extent and its involvement with neighboring structures such as the lung, pleura, mediastinum, and lymph nodes. Additionally, CT provides valuable information on the vascularity, composition, and density of the cancer lesion [15]. This comprehensive data is essential for accurate biopsy planning and guiding the treatment strategy.

3. <u>Magnetic Resonance Imaging (MRI)</u>: MRI assumes a crucial role in the diagnostic process, primarily due to its capacity to offer accurate tissue characterization and superior spatial resolution [15]. Beyond that, MRI aids in distinguishing chest-wall tumors from infectious or inflammatory processes, contributing valuable insights to biopsy planning [15]. In thoracic pathologies, MRI complements spiral CT and allows for contrast-media-free differentiation of solid tumors and vascular lesions, such as aortic aneurysms [2]. Its advantages become particularly apparent when multiplanar imaging is required before surgery to establish the exact spatial relationship between the tumor and other mediastinal structures [2]. This precise spatial information is invaluable for planning biopsy procedures and guiding subsequent therapeutic interventions.

4. <u>Positron Emission Tomography (PET/CT)</u>: FDG PET/CT serves as a complementary tool alongside conventional imaging methods when assessing mediastinal and chest wall masses [3]. It plays a vital role in disease staging and assessing treatment response, particularly in cases of sarcomas. The advantage of PET/CT lies

in its ability to provide functional information that complements the anatomical insights from other imaging modalities [3]. PET/CT's ability to pinpoint areas of interest more precisely can reduce the need for unnecessary invasive investigations. However, it's essential to note that even when PET/CT provides valuable insights, definitive diagnoses still require confirmatory tissue sampling to ensure accuracy [3].

Tumor Biopsy Outcomes:

The outcomes of core needle biopsies offer valuable insights into the diagnostic accuracy and adequacy of this procedure in the context of chest wall tumors. In a study analyzing 40 core needle biopsy samples, a critical distinction emerged: ten samples were from benign tumors, while the majority, comprising 30 samples, were from malignant tumors [4]. These findings underscore the importance of precise diagnostic tools for distinguishing between benign and malignant chest wall lesions.[4].

Diagnostic Accuracy of Core Needle Biopsy:

Benign vs. Malignant Tumors: One of the notable findings of this study was the discrepancy in diagnostic adequacy between core needle biopsies performed on benign and malignant tumors [4]. While core needle biopsy samples from malignant neoplasms displayed an impressive 83% adequacy rate, samples from benign tumors fell short with only 30% being deemed adequate [4]. This distinction highlights the diagnostic challenges posed by benign lesions and the need for additional diagnostic measures in such cases [4].

Nondiagnostic Samples:

Notably, many of the nondiagnostic samples obtained from benign lesions were associated with bony tumors, where 80% of such samples were inadequate [4]. In contrast, nondiagnostic samples from malignant sarcomas were largely from soft tissue tumors [4]. This suggests that the diagnostic yield of core needle biopsies may be impacted by the tumor's location, composition, and characteristics.[4].

Soft Tissue vs. Bony Sarcomas:

Examining the origin of the tumors provides further insights into the diversity of chest wall tumors. Out of 35 tumors evaluated, 54% were of soft tissue origin, while 43% were bony in nature [4]. Interestingly, in one case, a patient diagnosed with treatment-related sarcoma through core needle biopsy displayed a complete response to induction therapy, with no viable malignant cells found in the resection specimen upon pathologic examination [4]. This underscores the potential of core needle biopsy in guiding treatment decisions and assessing treatment response [4].

Comparative Advantages of Core Needle Biopsy:

Open surgical biopsies were regarded as the gold standard for diagnosing chest wall tumors [5]. However, this approach came with associated complications, including risks of seroma, infection, wound dehiscence, and tumor implantation [5]. Additionally, surgical biopsies incur the drawbacks of operating room time and cost, as well as the potential for inappropriately placed incisions that could compromise definitive resection or cosmesis [5].

Advantages of Image-Guided Core Needle Biopsies: Image-guided core needle biopsies have emerged as a viable alternative to open surgical biopsies in the context of chest wall tumors, offering accurate diagnostic results without the disadvantages of surgery, particularly in extremity cases [6-9]. While several studies have evaluated the efficacy of needle biopsies in chest wall lesions, they often encompassed a wide spectrum of malignancies, including carcinomas, benign tumors, and abscesses [6-9]. Consequently, limited reports exist specifically addressing the effectiveness of core needle biopsies in chest wall musculoskeletal tumors, particularly in the context of chest wall sarcomas [6-9].

Focus on Chest Wall Sarcomas: This study narrows its focus to the use of core needle biopsy in primary, metastatic, and recurrent sarcomas affecting the sternum, ribs, or soft tissues of the chest wall [6-9]. The study's primary objectives are twofold: (1) to evaluate the adequacy of tissue samples obtained through needle biopsy and (2) to assess the accuracy of this method in determining malignancy, histological subtype, and high-grade differentiation [6-9].

Impact of Tumor Characteristics: In this series, the majority of nondiagnostic samples from benign lesions were associated with bony tumors (4/5th), while nondiagnostic samples from malignant sarcomas primarily originated from soft tissue tumors [6, 13]. This discrepancy highlights the potential challenges associated with biopsying bony tumors, suggesting that cortex penetration might hinder the acquisition of adequate tissue samples [6, 13].

References:

1. Tateishi U, Gladish GW, Kusumoto M, Hasegawa T, Yokoyama R, Tsuchiya R, Moriyama N. Chest wall tumors: radiologic findings and pathologic correlation: part 2. Malignant tumors. Radiographics. 2003 Nov;23(6):1491-508.

2. Landwehr, P., Schulte, O. & Lackner, K. MR imaging of the chest: Mediastinum and chest wall. Eur Radiol 9, 1737–1744 (1999).

3. Tatci E, Ozmen O, Dadali Y, Biner IU, Gokcek A, Demirag F, Incekara F, Arslan N. The role of FDG PET/CT in evaluation of mediastinal masses and neurogenic tumors of chest wall. International journal of clinical and experimental medicine. 2015;8(7):11146

4. Kachroo P, Pak PS, Sandha HS, Nelson SD, Seeger LL, Cameron RB, Eilber FC, Lee JM. Chest wall sarcomas are accurately diagnosed by image-guided core needle biopsy. Journal of thoracic oncology. 2012 Jan 1;7(1):151-6

5. (Mankin HJ, Mankin CJ, Simon MA. The hazards of the biopsy, revisited. For the members of the Musculoskeletal Tumor Society. JBJS. 1996 May 1;78(5):656-3.)

6. Altuntas AO, Slavin J, Smith PJ, Schlict SM, Powell GJ, Ngan S, Toner G, Choong PF. Accuracy of computed tomography guided

core needle biopsy of musculoskeletal tumours. ANZ journal of surgery. 2005 Apr;75(4):187-91),

7. Hau M, Kim J, Kattapuram S, Hornicek FJ, Rosenberg AE, Gebhardt MC, Mankin HJ. Accuracy of CT-guided biopsies in 359 patients with musculoskeletal lesions. Skeletal radiology. 2002 Jun;31:349-53)

8. ssakov J, Flusser G, Koilender Y, Merimsky O, Lifschitz-Mercer B, Meller I. Computed tomography-guided core needle biopsy for bone and soft tissue tumors. IMAJ-RAMAT GAN-. 2003 Jan 1;5(1):28-30)

9. Logan PM, Connell DG, O'Connell JX, Munk PL, Janzen DL. Image-guided percutaneous biopsy of musculoskeletal tumors: an algorithm for selection of specific biopsy techniques. American Journal of Roentgenology. 1996 Jan 1;166:137-42.

10. Narvani AA, Tsiridis E, Saifuddin A, Briggs T, Cannon S. Does image guidance improve accuracy of core needle biopsy in diagnosis of soft tissue tumours?. Acta Orthopædica Belgica. 2009 Apr 1;75(2):239),

11. (Ray-Coquard I, Ranchere-Vince D, Thiesse P, Ghesquieres H, Biron P, Sunyach MP, Rivoire M, Lancry L, Méeus P, Sebban C, Blay JY. Evaluation of core needle biopsy as a substitute to open biopsy in the diagnosis of soft-tissue masses. European Journal of Cancer. 2003 Sep 1;39(14):2021-5),

12. (Soudack M, Nachtigal A, Vladovski E, Brook O, Gaitini D. Sonographically guided percutaneous needle biopsy of soft tissue masses with histopathologic correlation. Journal of Ultrasound in Medicine. 2006 Oct;25(10):1271-7.)

13. Hau M, Kim J, Kattapuram S, Hornicek FJ, Rosenberg AE, Gebhardt MC, Mankin HJ. Accuracy of CT-guided biopsies in 359 patients with musculoskeletal lesions. Skeletal radiology. 2002 Jun;31:349-53.)

14. (Thomas M, Shen KR. Primary tumors of the osseous chest wall and their management. Thoracic Surgery Clinics. 2017 May 1;27(2):181-93.)

15. (Bueno J, Lichtenberger III JP, Rauch G, Carter BW. MR imaging of primary chest wall neoplasms. Topics in Magnetic Resonance Imaging. 2018 Apr 1;27(2):83-93.

16. Kiatisevi P, Thanakit V, Sukunthanak B, Boonthatip M, Bumrungchart S, Witoonchart K. Computed tomography-guided core needle biopsy versus incisional biopsy in diagnosing musculoskeletal lesions. Journal of Orthopaedic Surgery. 2013 Aug;21(2):204-8

Chapter 6
Chest-Wall Tumor Management

Shubhajeet Roy, Md Kaif Khan, Dr Anurag Rai

Introduction:

Managing chest wall tumors is a multifaceted and interdisciplinary approach that encompasses the diagnosis, treatment, and care of individuals with various growths affecting the chest wall, which can be either benign or malignant. These tumors put unique challenges due to their location and potential impact on vital organs like the heart and lungs. Effective management often necessitates a collaborative approach involving surgeons, oncologists, radiologists, and other specialists to optimize patient outcomes. In this introduction, we will delve into the critical aspects of chest wall tumor treatment and management, considering the wide spectrum of clinical presentations and available treatment choices.

The management of chest-wall tumors hinges on an intricate interplay of factors encompassing tumor location, size, histology, stage, patient age, and comorbidities [1]. In this multifaceted landscape, the primary approach often involves surgical resection of the tumor, potentially followed by prosthetic reconstruction [1]. However, it's essential to acknowledge that not all chest wall tumors are amenable to immediate surgical intervention [1]. Furthermore, the presence of metastases in the chest wall may necessitate a nuanced treatment approach that combines surgical resection with complementary strategies, such as neoadjuvant chemotherapy or radiotherapy [1].

Enhancing Survival and Quality of Life:

For cases involving chest-wall metastases, surgical resection emerges as a pivotal intervention capable of extending overall survival and enhancing the patient's quality of life [1]. This surgical approach, when meticulously executed, offers a potent means to address metastatic chest-wall tumors [1]. However, the decision to pursue surgical excision isn't universal, and its appropriateness hinges on the specific tumor type and its responsiveness to neoadjuvant chemotherapy. In particular, highly chemo-sensitive tumors like osteosarcoma, Ewing sarcoma, and rhabdomyosarcoma may benefit from preoperative chemotherapy, with surgical considerations tailored to the therapeutic response [1]. On the contrary, some chest-wall tumors, exemplified by solitary plasmacytoma and Langerhans Cell Histiocytosis, are better suited for medical treatment, obviating the need for surgical intervention [1].

Surgical Resection for Chest-Wall Tumors:

Surgical Objectives:

In addressing chest-wall tumors, the paramount surgical goals encompass ensuring comprehensive oncological resection while securing adequate disease-free margins. These objectives are pivotal for optimizing patient outcomes [1].

Resection Margin Significance:

Extensive research has demonstrated the critical role of resection margins in disease-free survival [1]. Notably, a study conducted at the Mayo Clinic found that the width of the resection margin profoundly impacts patient survival rates. Patients who underwent surgery with a 4 cm resection margin exhibited a commendable 5-year survival rate of 56%, compared to the significantly lower 29% survival rate observed in those with a mere 2 cm resection margin [2].

Full-Thickness Resection for High-Grade Malignancies:

In cases involving tumors with a high grade of malignancy, achieving oncological radicality necessitates a comprehensive approach [1]. This involves full-thickness surgical resection, encompassing muscle, bone, and potentially even skin [3]. Particularly aggressive tumor lesions, known for their propensity to spread along the periosteum, mandate the complete removal of adjacent bone structures, such as ribs or the sternum, without compromising respiratory function [1]. Moreover, due to the heightened risk of metastasis to the subperiosteum and adjacent structures, resection of the rib segments both above and below the tumor is generally recommended [1-6]. The surgical principle of 'en bloc' removal is paramount, encompassing any previous biopsy scar and any other involved tissues or structures, including soft tissue, pleura, lung, and diaphragm [1]. In some cases, video-assisted thoracic surgery (VATS) can be a valuable tool for assessing tumor extent and the involvement of neighboring mediastinal organs [1]. It's important to position the thoracoscope away from the lesion to mitigate the risk of tumor spreading [7]. In chest-wall tumors, especially those displaying high malignancy, a radical approach to removal remains essential, with no compromise on the extent of oncological resection due to concerns about chest wall defects and subsequent reconstruction [7]. Lindford et al. demonstrated the feasibility and safety of wide resection in selected cases of extensive chest-wall recurrence breast cancer [7].

Surgical Approach Currently Followed:

In our approach to surgical management of chest-wall tumors, we adopt a comprehensive strategy [1]. This involves a skin incision encompassing the tumor site, areas affected by cancer, and regions previously subjected to radiotherapy We perform a wide surgical excision, including the tumor-bearing ribs, ensuring a minimum resection margin of 3 cm [1]. Additionally, removal of the adjacent rib segments above and below the tumor is standard practice to secure adequate resection margins [8]. In our center, sternal tumors are managed with partial, subtotal, or total sternectomy, with the extent of resection tailored to the lesion's dimensions. In all cases, bilateral removal of adjacent sternocostal cartilages is carried out [9].

Surgical precision is paramount in the management of chest-wall tumors [1]. Achieving adequate resection margins and accounting for tumor histotype play pivotal roles in securing favorable disease-free outcomes [1]. These principles, complemented by meticulous surgical technique and adherence to established classifications, collectively guide effective surgical strategies in this complex clinical domain [1].

Surgical Reconstruction for Chest-Wall Tumors:

Indications for Reconstruction

In the realm of chest-wall tumor management, surgical reconstruction is often a crucial step to restore both structural and functional integrity [10]. However, there is currently no universal consensus or guidelines that comprehensively outline the indications for chest-wall reconstruction hence, surgical approaches often rely on the surgeon's experience and preferences [10].

Defect Size and Repair Necessity:

Typically, not all chest-wall defects require repair [11]. Smaller defects, those measuring less than 5 cm, or resections involving fewer than three ribs, often do not necessitate reconstructive procedures[11]. In such cases, soft tissue alone is usually sufficient to cover the chest-wall breach [11]. Similarly, subscapular and apico-posterior chest-wall defects up to 10 cm in size are often left unreconstructed, as the scapula and shoulder can provide adequate support and stiffness [6,10].

Indications for Reconstruction:

While the need for reconstruction varies, certain indications are widely accepted within the surgical community. These include:

- Chest-wall defects exceeding 5 cm in diameter or with a total area greater than 100 cm^2[12].

- Resection involving more than three ribs from the anterior chest wall[12].
- Removal of over four ribs from the posterior chest wall[12].
- In cases of posterior resections, reconstruction is advised below the fourth rib to prevent scapular entrapment [12].

Timing of Reconstruction:

The timing of chest-wall reconstruction depends on the extent of the resection and whether the defect is partial or full-thickness [4]. In the case of full-thickness resections, reconstruction is often performed during the same surgical procedure [4]. This approach is essential to restore structural skeletal integrity, safeguard vital organs, and preserve respiratory function [4]. The fear of reconstruction should not limit the extent of the resection, emphasizing the importance of comprehensive surgical planning and collaboration with professionals, such as plastic surgeons [4]. If the surgeon lacks the requisite expertise, referral to experienced centers is advisable [4].

Options for Reconstruction:

Chest-wall reconstruction offers several options, encompassing both soft-tissue coverage and prosthetic materials [11]. Surgeons have access to various prosthetic materials to restore the chest wall, including synthetic materials, alloplastic substances, and biologic materials [11].

Prosthetic Material:

The ideal material for chest-wall prosthetic reconstruction should possess specific characteristics [10]. It should be rigid enough to prevent paradoxical movements, malleable for ease of use, highly resistant to infection, biologically inert, radiolucent for diagnostic purposes, and cost-effective [10].

Choice of Material:

However, it's important to note that there's no universally ideal material [1]. Often, combinations of these materials are employed. Each prosthetic material for reconstruction carries its own set of advantages and disadvantages [13-15]. Additionally, none has conclusively demonstrated superiority over others. Consequently, the choice of reconstruction method frequently hinges on the surgeon's preferences and expertise [13-15].

Synthetic Materials for Chest-Wall Reconstruction:

Flexible Synthetic Materials:

When it comes to chest-wall reconstruction, surgeons have a variety of synthetic materials at their disposal. These materials can be broadly categorized as flexible and rigid, each offering distinct advantages [10].

Flexible Materials:

Flexible synthetic materials, exemplified by Vicryl and polypropylene meshes, are prized for their malleability [10]. They can be stretched evenly in all directions, ensuring a uniform distribution of tension along the edges of the chest wall defect [10]. Moreover, their permeable nature helps reduce the risk of seromas [10].

* Vicryl and polypropylene meshes are notable examples of flexible materials [1].

* They provide even elongation and balanced tension distribution [1].

* Permeability reduces the likelihood of seromas [1].

Polytetrafluoroethylene (PTFE):

Polytetrafluoroethylene (PTFE), another flexible prosthetic material, plays a role in achieving a secure, watertight closure[10,13]. While it's effective for repairing larger chest-wall defects, its use often necessitates the addition of soft-tissue coverage or a muscle flap

[10,13]. Notably, PTFE should be avoided in cases of infection, as it's contraindicated in such scenarios [10,13].

* PTFE offers flexibility and a watertight seal[10,13].

* Additional soft-tissue coverage or muscle flap may be required [10,13].

* Contraindicated in cases of infection [10,13].

Rigid Synthetic Materials

Methyl Methacrylate:

Rigid synthetic materials, represented by Methyl methacrylate, are used to restore chest-wall rigidity following extensive rib or sternal resections [10]. This material, a resin, is frequently employed alongside polypropylene meshes in a "sandwich technique [10]." Initially, a layer of polypropylene meshes is applied to cover the defect, followed by the use of a methyl methacrylate substitute [10]. Subsequently, a second layer of polypropylene is added to encase the methyl methacrylate, and as an exothermic reaction takes place, the resin hardens [10]. It's crucial to consider potential drawbacks, including the possibility that the rigidity of methyl methacrylate could contribute to pain and atelectasis [10]. Moreover, its lack of permeability may lead to seromas and wound infections [10].

* Methyl methacrylate restores chest-wall rigidity [14].

* It's used alongside polypropylene meshes in a "sandwich technique [14]."

* Potential complications include pain, atelectasis, seromas, and wound infection [14].

Bioprosthetic Materials in Chest-Wall Reconstruction:

Bioprosthetic materials have emerged as a significant advancement in the field of chest-wall reconstruction. Over the past two decades, various biological meshes have been developed using human (allograft) or animal (xenograft) tissues [11,16,17]. These decellularized biological meshes serve as sturdy scaffolds, promoting tissue growth and healing through gradual revascularization and remodeling bypatient's own tissues[11,16,17]. They offer additional benefits, such as the stimulation of mesenchymal stem cell differentiation in the bone marrow and a 66% increase in fibroblast proliferation. Importantly, they exhibit remarkable resistance to infections, and some exist their removal even in cases that argue the age of infection [11 16,17].

Preferred Use of Biological Prosthetic Material:

1. Excellent Tissue Integration: Biological meshes like porcine dermis seamlessly integrate with surrounding tissues [1].

2. Ease of Placement: They are straightforward and quick to position [1].

3. Effective Fixation: They can be securely fastened under tension to the edges of the defect, enhancing stability [1].

Advantages Over Synthetic Materials:

Compared to synthetic materials, biological prostheses present several advantages, including a notable resistance to infections [1]. Synthetic materials carry the risk of complications, primarily due to their status as foreign bodies [1]. In our experience, we have encountered scenarios necessitating redo-surgeries, often involving the removal of infected synthetic meshes [1]. For substantial anterior chest-wall defects, we commonly combine biological prostheses with rigid systems, such as titanium bars, and myocutaneous flaps to bolster the reconstruction [1].

The Value of Biological Materials in Chest-Wall Reconstruction:

The reconstruction of the chest wall remains a formidable challenge [1]. It is firmly believed that biological materials offer a compelling alternative, especially in situations involving infected fields or patients at high risk of infection[1]. Additionally, biological meshes contribute to robust wound healing and long-term stability, with minimal postoperative complications [9]. Importantly, they are also deemed safe for use in pediatric patients [9].

Osteosynthesis Systems for Chest-Wall Reconstruction:

Osteosynthesis systems play a pivotal role in restoring the structural integrity of the chest wall, preventing paradoxical inward movements, prolonging mechanical ventilation, and minimizing chest-wall deformities while achieving favorable cosmetic outcomes [1]. They are primarily employed for stabilization and fixation following rib or sternum resection, including rib-to-sternum fixation and rib-to-rib fixation across the sternum [1]. The prevailing osteosynthesis systems in use today include STRATOS and MatrixRIB fixation [1]. These systems are constructed from titanium, a prosthetic material renowned for its high biocompatibility, inert nature, and compatibility with MRI scans [1]. Typically, they are employed in conjunction with biological or synthetic meshes, with or without the incorporation of myocutaneous flaps [11].

Titanium-Based Osteosynthesis Systems: A Preferred Choice

Numerous authors advocate for the superiority of titanium-based osteosynthesis systems, particularly in cases requiring the reconstruction of large full-thickness defects [1]. These systems have demonstrated a remarkable track record with few complications, including infections, bar fractures, or dislocations [9,18].

Surgical Procedures and Margin Considerations:

- Incision: Starting with an incision encompassing prior biopsy sites, invaded skin, and irradiated tissues [1].

- Margins: Maintaining a 3 cm margin around the tumor, removing adjacent ribs [1].

- Posterior Tumors: In some cases, resecting vertebral transverse processes for clear margins [1].

Benefits of Large Defect Reconstruction:

Reconstruction stabilizes the chest wall, reducing ventilation needs, preventing paradoxical chest-wall movements, and safeguarding vital organs [1].

Size-Based Reconstruction

Defects <5 cm (any location) or up to 10 cm (posterior) don't require reconstruction [19].

Diverse Reconstruction Materials:

Options include rigid and semi-rigid synthetic meshes (e.g., methyl-methacrylate and polytetrafluoroethylene), biocompatible prostheses (e.g., acellular dermal matrix), and titanium-based components [1]. The material choice depends on surgeon preference and patient-specific needs [1].

Advancements in Materials and 3D Printing:

New materials like cryopreserved homografts and allografts offer alternatives. 3D printing aids customized prosthesis creation, enhancing surgical planning [1].

3D-Printed Titanium Implant

We achieved a breakthrough by employing a 3D-printed titanium implant for a total sternectomy in a metastatic breast cancer patient[9]. This custom-made prosthesis, combined with a latissimus dorsi muscle flap, preserves rib-cage function, exemplifying our commitment to advancing chest-wall tumor surgery [9].

References:

1. Gonfiotti A, Salvicchi A, Voltolini L. Chest-Wall Tumors and Surgical Techniques: State-of-the-Art and Our Institutional Experience. Journal of Clinical Medicine. 2022 Sep 20;11(19):5516.

2. King RM, Pairolero PC, Trastek VF, Piehler JM, Payne WS, Bernatz PE. Primary chest wall tumors: factors affecting survival. The Annals of thoracic surgery. 1986 Jun 1;41(6):597-601.

3. Hazel K, Weyant MJ. Chest wall resection and reconstruction: management of complications. Thoracic surgery clinics. 2015 Nov 1;25(4):517-21.

4. Incarbone, MD M, Pastorino, MD U. Surgical treatment of chest wall tumors. World journal of surgery. 2001 Feb;25:218-30.

5. Shah AA, D'Amico TA. Primary chest wall tumors. Journal of the American College of Surgeons. 2010 Mar 1;210(3):360-6.

6. Thomas M, Shen KR. Primary tumors of the osseous chest wall and their management. Thoracic Surgery Clinics. 2017 May 1;27(2):181-93.

7. Lindford AJ, Jahkola TA, Tukiainen E. Late results following flap reconstruction for chest wall recurrent breast cancer. Journal of plastic, reconstructive & aesthetic surgery. 2013 Feb 1;66(2):165-73.

8. Gonfiotti A, Viggiano D, Vokrri E, Lucchi M, Divisi D, Crisci R, Mucilli F, Venuta F, Voltolini L. Chest wall reconstruction with implantable cross-linked porcine dermal collagen matrix: Evaluation of clinical outcomes. JTCVS techniques. 2022 Jun 1;13:250-60.

9. Bongiolatti S, Voltolini L, Borgianni S, Borrelli R, Innocenti M, Menichini G, Politi L, Tancredi G, Viggiano D, Gonfiotti A. Short and long-term results of sternectomy for sternal tumours. Journal of thoracic disease. 2017 Nov;9(11):4336.

10. Seder CW, Rocco G. Chest wall reconstruction after extended resection. Journal of thoracic disease. 2016 Nov;8(Suppl 11):S863.

11. Khullar OV, Fernandez FG. Prosthetic reconstruction of the chest wall. Thoracic Surgery Clinics. 2017 May 1;27(2):201-8.

12. Ito T, Suzuki H, Yoshino I. Mini review: surgical management of primary chest wall tumors. General thoracic and cardiovascular surgery. 2016 Dec;64:707-14.

13. Sanna S, Brandolini J, Pardolesi A, Argnani D, Mengozzi M, Dell'Amore A, Solli P. Materials and techniques in chest wall reconstruction: a review. Journal of visualized surgery. 2017;3.

14. Weyant MJ, Bains MS, Venkatraman E, Downey RJ, Park BJ, Flores RM, Rizk N, Rusch VW. Results of chest wall resection and reconstruction with and without rigid prosthesis. The Annals of thoracic surgery. 2006 Jan 1;81(1):279-85.

15. Deschamps C, Tirnaksiz BM, Darbandi R, Trastek VF, Allen MS, Miller DL, Arnold PG, Pairolero PC. Early and long-term results of prosthetic chest wall reconstruction. The Journal of thoracic and cardiovascular surgery. 1999 Mar 1;117(3):588-92.

16. Hoganson DM, O'Doherty EM, Owens GE, Harilal DO, Goldman SM, Bowley CM, Neville CM, Kronengold RT, Vacanti JP. The retention of extracellular matrix proteins and angiogenic and mitogenic cytokines in a decellularized porcine dermis. Biomaterials. 2010 Sep 1;31(26):6730-7.

17. Wiegmann B, Zardo P, Dickgreber N, Länger F, Fegbeutel C, Haverich A, Fischer S. Biological materials in chest wall reconstruction: initial experience with the Peri-Guard Repair Patch®. European journal of cardio-thoracic surgery. 2010 Mar 1;37(3):602-5.

18. Enneking WF, Spanier SS, Goodman MA. A system for the surgical staging of musculoskeletal sarcoma. Clinical

Orthopaedics and Related Research (1976-2007). 1980 Nov 1;153:106-20.

19. Gonfiotti A, Santini PF, Campanacci D, Innocenti M, Ferrarello S, Caldarella A, Janni A. Malignant primary chest-wall tumours: techniques of reconstruction and survival. European journal of cardio-thoracic surgery. 2010 Jul 1;38(1):39-45.

Chapter 7
Multidisciplinary Care and Team Approach

Shubhajeet Roy, Divya, Dr Shiv Rajan

Introduction:

Managing cancer patients on a global scale presents a formidable challenge due to the rapid evolution of clinical evidence, the continuous approval of new drugs, and frequent updates to scientific guidelines. Therefore a multidisciplinary approach towards cancer management is the need of the hour.

Definition of Multidisciplinary Team (MDT):

A multidisciplinary team (MDT) consists of a group of healthcare professionals from diverse disciplines, each contributing specific expertise to ensure that the patient receives comprehensive care and support [1].

Tumor Board Definition and Function:

In the National Cancer Institute's dictionary, a tumor board (or review) is defined as

A treatment planning approach in which a number of doctors who are experts in different specialties (disciplines) review and discuss the medical condition and treatment options of a patient [7].

Composition of Core and Non-Core Teams:

In the context of a Multidisciplinary Tumor Board (MTB), the "core team" typically consists of oncologists, surgeons specializing in various subspecialties, pathologists, radiotherapists, and other specialists chosen based on the specific cancer type being addressed [4,5,6].

The "non-core team" may encompass palliative-care physicians, medical students, psychologists, physicians in training, nursing staff specialists, research nurses, and coordinators.

The inclusion of members in the non-core team depends on regional practices and considerations [4,5,6]. In some countries, nurses play a pivotal role in influencing treatment decisions and are thus included in the core team rather than the non-core team [4,5,6].

Significance of MDT in Cancer Care:

The pivotal role of MDTs in cancer care was underscored by the 1995 Calman-Heine report, which recommended the establishment of arrangements for non-surgical oncological input into services, with a role for non-surgical oncologists and appointment of lead clinicians with a profound interest in cancer care within every Cancer Unit for organization and coordination of the range range of cancer services offered within the cancer unit [1].

Expanding Role Across Medical Specialties:

The growing emphasis on MDT management of cancer patients extends to encompass a wider array of medical specialties. Beyond surgeons and medical oncologists, this collaborative approach now includes general practitioners, pathologists, radiologists, palliative care specialists, and psychiatrists [3].

Recognizing the evolving landscape, it has become essential for medical students to gain early exposure to multidisciplinary principles and practices during their medical education. This early exposure fosters interdisciplinary interactions and the development of effective teamwork skills [3].

Interestingly, some forward-looking studies suggest that in the future, cancer patients themselves may actively participate in MDT meetings, reflecting a more patient-centered approach to care [3].

Physical and Virtual Multidisciplinary Approaches:

Multidisciplinary approaches traditionally involve physical meetings where specialists converge in the same location to collaboratively discuss clinical cases. However, the advancement of technology has given rise to virtual meetings, allowing physicians from different locations to engage in discussions and make the right diagnostic and therapeutic decisions effectively [8].

Molecular Tumor Boards (MTBs):

A specialized type of MDT is known as Molecular Tumor Boards (MTBs). The need to add to the "standard" MTB team a number of specialists focused on molecular biology has been felt due to the increasing use of molecular biology as a tool for supporting various therapeutic decisions. This board typically includes pathologists, oncologists, hematologists, basic scientists, and genetic counselors [4].

MTBs utilize genetic cancer-cell profiling to predict a patient's response to drug sensitivity and resistance. Also, the molecular board takes into account clinical factors and targetable genetic alterations and provides the clinician with the best possible treatment options. This personalized approach ensures optimal treatment strategies based on individual patient profiles [4].

Benefits of MTBs:

MTBs offer a multitude of advantages for patients, physicians, the community, and hospitals, including

1. Ensuring uniformity in standards of care for cancer patients.
2. Facilitating open communication channels for the exchange of scientific evidence, guidelines, and experiential knowledge among physicians.
3. Providing mechanisms for reviewing the quality of professional care.
4. Considering patient demographics, comorbidities, preferences, and social support, which are often overlooked in clinical guidelines.
5. Enhancing decision-making processes, improving the presentation of medical information, and promoting effective teamwork within the medical community [9-12].

Challenges in Global cancer care:

While it is well-established that MDTs generally enhance patient outcomes, several barriers hinder their full realization. These barriers include limitations in facilities, time constraints, and challenges in building strong interprofessional relationships [1].

Furthermore, studies have revealed instances where decisions made during MDT meetings may not always translate effectively into practice [2].

References-
1. Whitehouse M. A policy framework for commissioning cancer services. BMJ. 1995 Jun 3;310(6992):1425-6.
2. Blazeby JM, Wilson L, Metcalfe C, Nicklin J, English R, Donovan JL. Analysis of clinical decision-making in multi-disciplinary cancer teams. Annals of Oncology. 2006 Mar 1;17(3):457-60.
3. Choy ET, Chiu A, Butow P, Young J, Spillane A. A pilot study to evaluate the impact of involving breast cancer patients in the multidisciplinary discussion of their disease and treatment plan. The Breast. 2007 Apr 1;16(2):178-89.
4. El Saghir NS, Keating NL, Carlson RW, Khoury KE, Fallowfield L. Tumor boards: optimizing the structure and improving efficiency of multidisciplinary management of patients with cancer worldwide. American Society of Clinical Oncology Educational Book. 2014 Jan 1;34(1):e461-6.
5. Hermes-Moll K, Dengler R, Riese C, Baumann W. Tumor boards from the perspective of ambulant oncological care. Oncology Research and Treatment. 2016 May 25;39(6):377-83.
6. Lumenta DB, Sendlhofer G, Pregartner G, Hart M, Tiefenbacher P, Kamolz LP, Brunner G. Quality of teamwork in multidisciplinary cancer team meetings: A feasibility study. PloS one. 2019 Feb 15;14(2):e0212556.
7. Berardi R, Morgese F, Rinaldi S, Torniai M, Mentrasti G, Scortichini L, Giampieri R. Benefits and limitations of a multidisciplinary approach in cancer patient management. Cancer Management and Research. 2020 Sep 30:9363-74.
8. Takeda T, Takeda S, Uryu K, Ichihashi Y, Harada H, Iwase A, Tamura Y, Hibino M, Horiuchi S, Kani H. Multidisciplinary lung cancer tumor board connecting eight general hospitals in Japan via a high-security communication line. JCO Clinical Cancer Informatics. 2019 Mar;3:1-7.

9. Croke JM, El-Sayed S. Multidisciplinary management of cancer patients: chasing a shadow or real value? An overview of the literature. Current Oncology. 2012 Aug;19(4):232-8.

10. Gross GE. The role of the tumor board in a community hospital. CA: a cancer journal for clinicians. 1987 Mar 1;37(2):88-92.

11. Somashekhar SP, Sepúlveda MJ, Puglielli S, Norden AD, Shortliffe EH, Kumar CR, Rauthan A, Kumar NA, Patil P, Rhee K, Ramya Y. Watson for Oncology and breast cancer treatment recommendations: agreement with an expert multidisciplinary tumor board. Annals of Oncology. 2018 Feb 1;29(2):418-23.

12. Lamb BW, Green JS, Benn J, Brown KF, Vincent CA, Sevdalis N. Improving decision making in multidisciplinary tumor boards: prospective longitudinal evaluation of a multicomponent intervention for 1,421 patients. Journal of the American College of Surgeons. 2013 Sep 1;217(3):412-20.

Chapter 8
Research and Advancements:

Shubhajeet Roy, Divyansh Ahuja, Prof Vijay Kumar

Introduction:

In 1906, Dr. Tansini pioneered chest wall reconstruction by employing a pedicled latissimus dorsi flap to address anterior chest wall defects [1]. Since then, the field of chest wall reconstruction has undergone a remarkable evolution, driven by advances in surgical techniques and the availability of diverse prosthetic and bioprosthetic materials [2]. Unfortunately, extensive chest wall resections have historically led to considerable morbidity and limited patients' ability to perform daily activities [3,4]. However, the relentless progress in surgical methodologies, postoperative care, and rehabilitation has significantly reduced perioperative complications and mortality rates [15]. Collaboration across multiple medical disciplines, including thoracic surgeons, plastic surgeons, neurosurgeons, and medical and radiation oncologists, remains paramount for optimal patient outcomes [15].

Innovations in Allograft and Homograft Technique:

The evolution of allograft and homograft techniques has introduced novel approaches to restore chest wall structural stability [9]. Notably, the utilization of cryopreserved allografts and homografts, sourced from cadaveric donors and stored at subzero temperatures, has gained prominence for addressing large chest wall defects [5,6]. These materials exhibit variations in cytotoxicity, bacterial adhesion, and biomechanical properties compared to conventional prosthetics, offering unique advantages [7]. Emerging materials like titanium plates, cryopreserved grafts, and acellular collagen matrices are increasingly adopted in chest wall reconstruction, providing enhanced incorporation, structural stability, and reduced susceptibility to infection [8].

Advanced Techniques for Complex Defects:

Innovations such as the arena roof technique have emerged as effective strategies to tackle extensive chest wall defects, involving a combination of prosthetic or bioprosthetic materials and the use of titanium plates and a cellular collagen matrix have enhanced the selection capabilities of materials used for complex chest wall construction [8]. Also in order to restore chest wall continuity and function use of biomimetic reconstruction is widely accepted [13].

Transition to Synthetic Meshes

The historical use of metal prostheses has given way to synthetic meshes, with methyl methacrylate, strategically placed between mesh layers, emerging as the preferred choice since the 1980s [10]. The introduction of titanium plates represents a significant milestone, capitalizing on their corrosion resistance, lightweight nature, impressive tensile strength, compatibility with MRI, and crucial biocompatibility [10]. Pioneering the use of sternal ceramic prostheses, like Ceratite, offers notable benefits in terms of osteoconductivity, strength, and biocompatibility, and eliminates the risk of disease transmission associated with certain materials [11]. Additionally, the Ley prosthesis, constructed from titanium, has been increasingly employed for stabilizing the sternum following postoperative mediastinitis and sternal dehiscence [12].

Advancements in Managing Chest Wall Tumors (Advancements in surgical approach):

The refinement of modern surgical techniques for managing chest wall tumors traces back to the 1960s and 1970s, contributing significantly to improved morbidity and mortality rates [14].Resection stands as the primary treatment modality for chest wall tumors. Earlier open thoracotomy was the approach for chest wall resection however it is significantly associated with post-operative pain and morbidity. Depending on the location and size of the defect, chest wall reconstruction is often necessary to safeguard underlying structures, maintain respiratory mechanics, and reduce respiratory complications [22].

The arrival of minimally invasive techniques like (VATS) video-assisted thoracic surgery and robotic thoracic surgery offer potential advantages over open thoracotomy by reducing post-operative mortality [23]. These benefits cover smaller incisions, avoidance of rib spreading, preservation of uninvolved overlying major muscles, minimized tissue trauma, reduced inflammatory response, decreased postoperative pain, shorter hospital stays, and quicker recovery [24].

Also, advancements in methods of flap reconstruction, coupled with improvements in intensive care and rehabilitation, have played pivotal roles in these positive outcomes [15].

Imaging Techniques:

The past half-century has witnessed remarkable developments in various imaging modalities, including computed tomography (CT), positron emission tomography (PET), magnetic resonance imaging (MRI), single-photon emission computed tomography (SPECT), digital mammography, and sonography.These advanced medical imaging techniques have matured and assumed essential roles in patient management and diagnostic processes.

Future Innovations:

Despite recent progress in variable-angle titanium prosthetic bar design, opportunities for enhancement remain [16]. Future chest wall prostheses are pdesigned to become highly personalized, with shape and size tailored to individual patients. Also, the emergence of three-dimensional printing and rapid prototyping has significantly influenced the field of reconstructive surgery, particularly in dealing with intricate challenges involving extensive areas of the body [17]. Surgeons often face complex situations when dealing with the thorax, abdomen, or limbs due to the intricate structures and various pathologies involved. Three-dimensional printing technology has progressively improved its ability to replicate these structures with remarkable accuracy. As a result, it has become an invaluable tool for healthcare professionals, helping them not only in the pre-surgical planning stage but also during the actual surgical procedures [17].

Incorporating Regenerative Techniques:

The adoption of hybrid operating rooms equipped with real-time cone-beam computed tomography has gained prominence in thoracic surgery, offering enhanced procedural accuracy [19]. Pioneering work by Metcalfe and Ferguson suggests that a combination of biomaterials, wound healing processes, embryonic development principles, stem cell therapies, and regeneration techniques could potentially replace all skin layers [20]. The investigation of biodegradable materials such as collagen-coated polydioxanone and polycaprolactone is ongoing.Tissue engineering of the skin aims to achieve complete regeneration, encompassing skin appendages, layers (epidermis, dermis, and fatty subcutus), vascularization, and the establishment of functional vascular and nerve networks, leading to scar-free integration with surrounding host tissue [20]. Furthermore, bone marrow mesenchymal stem cells (BMSCs) are emerging as an ideal cell source for bone tissue engineering. Combining BMSCs with polydioxanone mesh holds promise for replacing ribs and facilitating the reconstruction of relatively small chest wall defects [21].

References:

1. Tansini I. Sopra il mio nuovo processo di amputazione della mammella. Gazz Med Ital. 1906;57(57):141.

2. Seder CW, Rocco G. Chest wall reconstruction after extended resection. Journal of thoracic disease. 2016 Nov;8(Suppl 11):S863.

3. Geissen NM, Medairos R, Davila E, Basu S, Warren WH, Chmielewski GW, Liptay MJ, Arndt AT, Seder CW. Number of ribs resected is associated with respiratory complications following lobectomy with en bloc chest wall resection. Lung. 2016 Aug;194:619-24.

4. Daigeler A, Druecke D, Hakimi M, Duchna HW, Goertz O, Homann HH, Lehnhardt M, Steinau HU. Reconstruction of the thoracic wall—long-term follow-up including pulmonary function tests. Langenbeck's archives of surgery. 2009 Jul;394:705-15.

5. Seder CW, Rocco G. Chest wall reconstruction after extended resection. Journal of thoracic disease. 2016 Nov;8(Suppl 11):S863.

6. Ng CS. Recent and future developments in chest wall reconstruction. InSeminars in thoracic and cardiovascular surgery 2015 Jun 1 (Vol. 27, No. 2, pp. 234-239). WB Saunders.

7. Wiegmann B, Korossis S, Burgwitz K, Hurschler C, Fischer S, Haverich A, Kuehn C. In vitro comparison of biological and synthetic materials for skeletal chest wall reconstruction. The Annals of Thoracic Surgery. 2015 Mar 1;99(3):991-8.

8. Rocco G, La Rocca A, La Manna C, Martucci N, De Luca G, Accardo R. Arena roof technique for complex reconstruction after extensive chest wall resection. The Annals of Thoracic Surgery. 2015 Oct 1;100(4):1479-81.

9. Gangolphe L, Tixier L. Enorme enchondrome de la fourchette sternale. Lyon Chir. 1909;2:112.

10. Sanna S, Brandolini J, Pardolesi A, Argnani D, Mengozzi M, Dell'Amore A, Solli P. Materials and techniques in chest wall reconstruction: a review. Journal of visualized surgery. 2017;3.

11. Watanabe A, Watanabe T, Obama T, Ohsawa H, Mawatari T, Ichimiya Y, Takahashi N, Abe T. New material for reconstruction of the anterior chest wall, including the sternum. The Journal of Thoracic and Cardiovascular Surgery. 2003 Oct 1;126(4):1212-4.

13. Pedersen TA, Pilegaard HK. Reconstruction of the thorax with Ley prosthesis after resection of the sternum. The Annals of Thoracic Surgery. 2009 Apr 1;87(4):e31-3.

14. Rocco G. Chest wall resection and reconstruction according to the principles of biomimesis. InSeminars in Thoracic and Cardiovascular Surgery 2011 Dec 1 (Vol. 23, No. 4, pp. 307-313). WB Saunders.

15. Tukiainen E, Popov P, Asko-Seljavaara S. Microvascular reconstructions of full-thickness oncological chest wall defects. Annals

16. Seder CW, Rocco G. Chest wall reconstruction after extended resection. Journal of thoracic disease. 2016 Nov;8(Suppl 11):S863.

17. Hussain S, Mubeen I, Ullah N, Shah SS, Khan BA, Zahoor M, Ullah R, Khan FA, Sultan MA. Modern diagnostic imaging technique applications and risk factors in the medical field: A review. BioMed Research International. 2022 Jun 6;2022.

18. Young JS, McAllister M, Marshall MB. Three-dimensional technologies in chest wall resection and reconstruction. Journal of Surgical Oncology. 2023 Feb;127(2):336-42.

19. Di Rosa L. 3D Printing for Whole Body Reconstruction. In3D Printing in Plastic Reconstructive and Aesthetic Surgery: A Guide for Clinical Practice 2022 Sep 20 (pp. 85-90). Cham: Springer International Publishing.

20. Schroeder C, Chung JM, Mitchell AB, Dillard TA, Radaelli AG, Schampaert S. Using the hybrid operating room in thoracic surgery: a paradigm shift. Innovations. 2018 Sep;13(5):372-7.

21. Metcalfe AD, Ferguson MW. Tissue engineering of replacement skin: the crossroads of biomaterials, wound healing, embryonic development, stem cells and regeneration. Journal of the Royal Society Interface. 2007 Jun 22;4(14):413-37.

22. Tang H, Xu Z, Qin X, Wu B, Wu L, Zhao X, Li Y. Chest wall reconstruction in a canine model using polydioxanone mesh, demineralized bone matrix and bone marrow stromal cells. Biomaterials. 2009 Jul 1;30(19):3224-33.

23. Leuzzi G, Nachira D, Cesario A, Novellis P, Petracca Ciavarella L, Lococo F, Facciolo F, Granone P, Margaritora S. Chest wall tumors and prosthetic reconstruction: A comparative analysis on functional outcome. Thoracic cancer. 2015 May;6(3):247-54.

24. Verm RA, Vigneswaran WT, Lin A, Zywiciel J, Freeman R, Abdelsattar ZM. Robotic chest wall resection for primary benign chest wall tumors and locally advanced lung cancer: an institutional case series and national report. Journal of Thoracic Disease. 2023 Sep 28;15(9).

25. Dal Agnol G, Oliveira R, Ugalde PA. Video-assisted thoracoscopic surgery lobectomy with chest wall resection. Journal of Thoracic Disease. 2018 Aug;10(Suppl 22):S2656.

Chapter 9
Resource and Support for Patients

Divya, Mehul Saxena, Dr Anurag Rai, Prof Parijat Suryavanshi

Introduction:

Dealing with chest wall tumors can be challenging, and a supportive network is invaluable. Support groups come in online and local formats, each with unique benefits. Online groups provide virtual connections and information but may have challenges like miscommunication and anonymity. Local groups offer face-to-face interactions, creating a sense of community. However, specific chest wall tumor support groups can be scarce due to the condition's rarity.

In the absence of dedicated support groups, patients and caregivers can turn to general cancer support groups and online communities. These platforms offer emotional support and shared experiences. Always inform your healthcare provider about your participation in a support group to ensure comprehensive medical care. Support and resources are essential in navigating the complexities of chest wall tumors.

Support Groups for Chest Wall Tumors:

- Support groups play a crucial role in providing emotional support, sharing knowledge, and offering practical assistance to individuals affected by chest wall tumors [4].

- They serve as a valuable resource for patients, their families, and caregivers who are navigating the challenges of this condition.
- Support groups come in two primary formats - online and local. Each offers unique benefits:

Online Support Groups:

- Online support groups provide a platform for individuals to connect, exchange experiences, and access information related to chest wall tumors [1].
- These groups can be particularly helpful for patients and caregivers who might not have easy access to local, face-to-face support groups.
- However, it's important to be aware of some potential challenges associated with online groups:
- Written text communication can sometimes lead to misunderstandings or confusion among group members.
- Anonymity may encourage some participants to make inappropriate comments or engage in disrespectful behaviors.
- Excessive online participation can unintentionally isolate individuals from their friends and family.
- Online communities can also be susceptible to misinformation or information overload [1].

Local Support Groups:

- Local support groups offer a physical, face-to-face setting where individuals dealing with chest wall tumors can come together.
- These groups create a sense of community and provide a platform for immediate, personal interactions.
- Participants often find comfort in meeting others who share similar experiences.

Post-Treatment Guidance for Chest Wall Tumors

- After undergoing treatment for chest wall tumors, it's essential to follow a prescribed post-treatment plan [2].
- Patient's healthcare provider will guide him/her through the recovery process, including follow-up appointments.
- Here are specific aspects of post-treatment guidance that one may need to consider:

Activity Restrictions:

- The healthcare provider will provide guidance on any activity restrictions, ensuring a safe and smooth recovery process.

Chest Physiotherapy:

- Chest physiotherapy involves a set of exercises designed to help you regain your strength and facilitate the healing process.

Surgical Wound Care:

- If the treatment involves surgery, proper care of your surgical wound is crucial for avoiding complications.

Support Groups for Chest Wall Tumors - A Unique Challenge

- Unlike some more common medical conditions, specific support groups exclusively dedicated to chest wall tumors may not always be readily available.
- The unique nature of chest wall tumors, coupled with their relative rarity, can result in the absence of condition-specific support groups.

Alternative Resources and Support for Chest Wall Tumor Patients

- In the absence of dedicated chest wall tumor support groups, patients and their caregivers have alternative resources and support options:

General Cancer Support Groups:

- Seek support from general cancer support groups that address a broad range of topics related to various cancer types. While not condition-specific, these groups can provide emotional support, shared experiences, and practical advice.

Online Communities:

- Explore online communities dedicated to cancer patients. These platforms offer a space for individuals affected by various forms of cancer to connect and share their experiences. They can be a valuable resource for chest wall tumor patients.

- Keep in mind that while support groups offer emotional and informational support, they should complement rather than replace regular medical care.

- Always inform your healthcare provider about your participation in a support group to ensure that you receive comprehensive medical attention [3].

References:

1. Information on Thoracic Support Groups: https://scts.org/patients/support_groups/thoracic_support_groups.aspx

2. Post-Treatment Information for Chest Wall Tumors: https://my.clevelandclinic.org/health/diseases/23482-chest-wall-tumor

3. Support Groups and Their Role in Coping: https://www.mayoclinic.org/healthy-lifestyle/stress-management/in-depth/support-groups/art-20044655

4. Graper ML, Schilsky ML. The Role of Patient Support Groups in Managing Wilson Disease. Handbook of Clinical Neurology. 2017 Jan 1;142:231-40.

About the Book

Discover a comprehensive exploration of chest wall tumors in our detailed book catered to healthcare professionals, caregivers and patients covering the essentials of the diverse spectrum of chest wall tumor types.

This book is a vital resource offering a deep dive into chest wall tumors, explaining how they are diagnosed, treated, and managed. It's a reliable companion that educates and supports readers through the complexities of these tumors.

Written by medical professionals, this book is designed to support individuals affected by chest wall tumors, equipping them with vital knowledge to navigate their unique medical journey with confidence and understanding. It is a reliable and compassionate guide for anyone seeking a deeper understanding of chest wall tumors.

www.ingramcontent.com/pod-product-compliance
Lightning Source LLC
LaVergne TN
LVHW061618070526
838199LV00078B/7334